Nurse Management & Executive Practice

Nurse Management & Executive Practice

Al Rundio, PhD, DNP, RN, APRN, NEA-BC, FNAP, FIAAN, FAAN
Associate Dean for Academic Nursing
Chief Academic Nursing Officer
Clinical Professor of Nursing
Drexel University
College of Nursing & Health Professions
Philadelphia, Pennsylvania

Hospital Trustee
Inspira Health System
Mullica Hill, New Jersey

Wolters Kluwer

Philadelphia • Baltimore • New York • London
Buenos Aires • Hong Kong • Sydney • Tokyo

Acquisitions Editor: Nicole Dernoski
Marketing Manager: Linda Wetmore
Production Project Manager: Linda Van Pelt
Editorial Coordinator: Dave Murphy
Design Coordinator: Elaine Kasmer
Manufacturing Coordinator: Kathleen Brown
Prepress Vendor: TNQ Technologies

9 8 7 6 5 4 3 2 1

Printed in China

Library of Congress Cataloging-in-Publication Data

Names: Rundio, Al, editor.
Title: Nurse management and executive practice / [edited by] Al Rundio.
Description: Philadelphia, PA : Wolters Kluwer, [2019] | Includes bibliographic references and index.
Identifiers: LCCN 2018031107 | ISBN 9781496380913
Subjects: | MESH: Nurse Administrators | Nursing Services—organization & administration
Classification: LCC RT89 | NLM WY 105 | DDC 362.17/3068—dc23 LC record available at https://lccn.loc.gov/2018031107

shop.lww.com

CCS0918

DEDICATION

I dedicate this book to my two best friends, Luke and Logan. Logan is our 10-year-old Papillon dog. He has been extremely healthy all of his life. In fact, a vet recently told us that from his condition it looks like he is 4 years old. Luke is my 10-year-old Papillon. Luke has had an amazing life in that he has had several medical issues. He has pica, and in his first year he had 3 major surgeries to save his life. In the summer of 2017 he was diagnosed with liver failure and had a surgically correctable congenital liver shunt.

I also dedicate this book to the medical, nursing, professional, and support staffs of the Matthew J. Ryan Veterinary Hospital of the University of Pennsylvania in Philadelphia, Pennsylvania. This hospital has given Luke a second chance on life 4 times. The care at this world-renowned veterinary hospital is simply incredible. Luke gets far better care than what most human beings receive in human hospitals. If every human hospital adopted the quality metrics of the Matthew J. Ryan Veterinary Hospital of the University of Pennsylvania, we would not have major quality problems in our nation's hospitals. A special thank you to the following medical staff: Dr. Adreanne Cleroux-Gaboury, DVM, IPSAV, Internal Medicine; Dr. Stephen Cai, VMD, Internal Medicine; Dr. Rebecca Stevens, VMD, Internal Medicine;

Dr. Jennifer Huck, DVM, DACVS, Surgeon; Dr. Mary Dell Deweese, DVM, Surgeon. A special thanks to both Emily and Fantasia. Emily is a fourth-year veterinary student. She was on her internal medicine rotation when Luke was diagnosed. She gave us the great news that Luke had a correctable liver problem. Fantasia is a fourth-year veterinary student. She was on her surgical rotation. Her more than positive attitude made our decision to have Luke have surgery much easier.

A dog is the only thing on earth that loves you more than you love yourself.

—Josh Billings
(Read more at: https://www.brainyquote.com/quotes/keywords/dog.html)

You can tell by the kindness of a dog how a human should be.

—Captain Beefheart
(Read more at: https://www.brainyquote.com/quotes/keywords/dog.html)

Al Rundio

LUKE

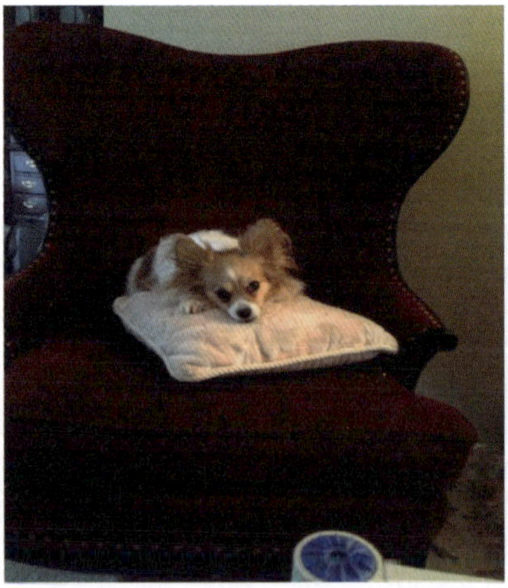

LOGAN

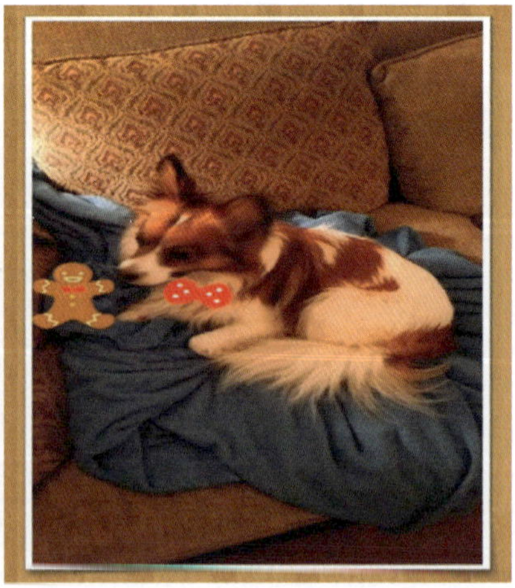

Contributors

Kathleen Bradbury-Golas, DNP, RN, FNP-C, ACNS-BC
Associate Clinical Professor
Nurse Practitioner Program
College of Nursing and Health Professions
Drexel University
Philadelphia, PA

Frances H. Cornelius PhD, MSN, RN-BC, CNE
Chair and Professor
Director of Quality, Safety and Risk Management in Healthcare Program
Coordinator of Clinical Informatics Education
Graduate Nursing and Complementary & Integrative Health Departments
College of Nursing and Health Professions
Drexel University
Philadelphia, PA

Mary Gallagher Gordon, Ph.D, MSN, RN, CNE
Associate Dean, Technology and Compliance
Associate Clinical Professor of Nursing
College of Nursing & Health Professions
Drexel University
Philadelphia, PA

William J. Lorman, JD, PhD, MSN
Assistant Clinical Professor
College of Nursing & Health Professions
Drexel University
Philadelphia, PA

Virginia "Ginny" Wilson, MSN, RN, NEA-BC, NE-BC
Director, Nursing Leadership in Health Services Management
Advanced Role MSN Program
Director, Innovation in Nursing
Advanced Role MSN Program
Assistant Professor
College of Nursing and Health Professions
Drexel University
Philadelphia, PA

Preface

Nurse executive practice has certainly changed and expanded over the years.

It is important to recognize that any nurse in a management position is an executive. This encompasses those nurse managers on the front line all the way up the ladder to the chief nursing officer/chief nursing executive.

Today, the nurse executive must have competency in various areas of practice. The American Organization of Nurse Executives (AONE) defines specific competencies of executive nursing practice. The competencies that a nurse executive must have are inclusive of but not limited to leadership, human capital management, research and evidence-based practice, data analysis, legal and ethical issues, strategic planning, communication skills, strategic partners, assessment of communities, promotion of health and prevention for patients, quality and patient safety, informatics, innovation, and fiscal management.

The nurse executive of today must be a visionary. A proactive stance to management is critical in today's business and health care environment.

Health care reform and managed care have led to the creation of new models of care as well as mergers and acquisitions of hospitals. More nurse executives will be leading at a corporate level over large health systems. More nurse executives may find themselves serving on hospital and other types of boards and commissions. There are many more practice environments today. Nurse executives will be needed in an array of different practices. Care is moving away from the hospital to other types of centers and services being offered in the community.

Education is also being transformed. More nurse executives will be prepared at the doctoral level, in particular, the Doctor of Nursing Practice (DNP) level. Secondary to the Magnet Recognition Program of the American Nurses Credentialing Center (ANCC), many more nurse executives will be board certified in executive practice.

The primary purpose of this book is to prepare nurse executives to successfully pass the nurse executive examinations offered by ANCC and AONE. When reviewing and reading this book, one should take note of what they know and, more important, what they do not know or what they are weak in. A program of study that focuses on the weakest areas of knowledge should be implemented. Each chapter has questions that can assist you in the preparation for these examinations.

I hope that you enjoy the book and that you find it helpful for your success and certification.

Al Rundio

Contents

CHAPTER

1

Leadership Responsibilities

Al Rundio and Kathleen Bradbury-Golas

This chapter will review:

LEADERSHIP THEORIES

ORGANIZATIONAL THEORIES

GOVERNANCE

BUSINESS MODELS

STRATEGIC PARTNERSHIPS

MODELS OF NURSING CARE

COMMUNICATION

CASE STUDIES

LEADERSHIP THEORY

There are many theories on leadership. This chapter will begin with a review of these theories.

Great Man Theory

The great man theory states that one is born a leader. In other words, one has leadership talent and skill as part of his or her makeup. Most likely individuals who have such talent have been socialized in an environment that prepares them for leadership. An example would be Prince William who has been mentored since birth to be a king. Today, most educators do not believe that one is born a leader. The belief is that one is educated to be a leader. Also paramount to this is what one is socialized to, as well as some of their innate traits for leadership.

Trait Theory

The premise of this theory is that a leader has many traits, for example, humor, visionary, collaboration, humanism, and intelligence.

Path-Goal Theory

This theory centers on attaining the organizational goals and objectives. The leader shows the subordinate the pathway on how to accomplish these goals.

Contingency Theory

Contingency theory consists of 3 variables: leader, power, and leader-subordinate relationships. The effectiveness of the leader centers on how these 3 variables interact. For example, I could be a wonderful leader, I could have excellent relationships with my subordinates, yet I have no power. Every time I make a decision I have to get approval from the chief executive officer (CEO). Thus, staff perceive my leadership style as ineffective because I cannot make decisions on my own. Another example would be that the leader has great power but the relationships with subordinates are poor, and therefore subordinates do not want to work in the organization. The best leader would have power, would be an excellent leader, and would have great relationships with his or her subordinates. This theory is one of the more important theories, as the concepts in this theory are testable.

Situational Theory

The premise of this leadership theory centers on the situation at hand. For example, I may be a leader who believes in participative management. However, when a patient has a cardiac arrest and the staff are not doing what they are supposed to do, I could become very autocratic and assign individuals task to make certain that the patient is resuscitated appropriately.

Life Cycle Theory

This theory is based on the work of Dr. Kenneth Blanchard. He has designed a leadership survey tool in which one completes the survey and then plots one's score in a 4-quadrant box. The top 2 quadrants are high task and high relationship; the bottom 2 quadrants are low task and low relationship. An ideal leader would have the qualities of high task and high relationship. This would certainly accomplish the organizational goals, and it also implies that the leader gets along well with subordinates. An autocrat would have high task and low relationship scores. This implies that the autocrat gets a lot accomplished through the fear factor. Blanchard found that most individuals score average for task accomplishment and relationship.

Transactional Theory

Transactional theory is based on Eric Berne's psychological theory. Berne examined how individuals deal with anxiety. The basic premise is that anxiety creates states in which individuals use defense mechanisms to control anxiety, because anxiety can lead to more psychotic states. One way to control anxiety is through medication. Berne's work was to use psychology and counseling to help the client see what is causing anxiety so that the cause can be eliminated or corrected. He described the interaction of the counselor with the client as a transaction; hence the term transactional analysis. Now how do we apply this to leadership? The transaction that occurs between a leader and a subordinate is to help the subordinate achieve the goals of the organization. Therefore transactional theory and leadership are very closely related to path-goal theory. Berne also said that we function in various roles, such as parent, adult, and child. When we observe human behavior in the organization, do we not see some of these roles at play?

Transformational Leadership Theory

The transformational leader is one who inspires and motivates others to succeed. This type of leader has the finger on the pulse but is not a micromanager. This leader encourages others to take risk. Should a person fail at a risk, this leader does not get upset but rather attributes this to a learning experience. In other words, without taking a risk, one would not achieve anything. This type of leader transforms the culture of an organization. The Magnet Recognition Program by the American Nurses Credentialing Center has at the core transformational leadership.

TRANSFORMATIONAL LEADERSHIP

Burns defined transformational leadership as a process in which "leaders and followers raise one another to higher levels of motivation and morality" (Burns, 1978, p. 21). It is based on empowering others to engage in pursuing a collective purpose by working together to achieve a vision of the preferred future. Both leader and follower are influenced and "transformed." It is important to remember that there are 2 types of leaders: the traditional manager concerned with the day-to-day operations (transactional leader) and the leader who is committed to a vision that empowers others (transformational leader). A good leader demonstrates both transactional and transformational characteristics.

Doody and Doody (2012) state that nurses have been overmanaged and led inadequately. Yet in today's society, with ever-increasing health care needs and changes, there are great opportunities for change. This will require more flexible leadership.

Transformational leaders are those who motivate their followers to do what must be done to reach or accomplish a shared goal. These leaders commit people to action, convert followers into leaders, and convert leaders into change agents. Effective transformational leaders identify themselves as change agents, are courageous, believe in people, are driven by values, love to learn, and are visionary. It does not matter what position a person holds within an organization—anyone who possesses those characteristics can transform it. At the organizational level, it is about innovation and change.

There are 4 characteristics needed to be a transformational leader:

1. ***Idealized influence***: Instead of being promoted according to seniority and having the ability to "conform" to all the rules and regulations, nurse leaders must be charming, be committed to a vision or goal, and manage staff accordingly. This vision or goal should be not only an organization's goal but also one to which the leader aspires. This will often put the leader in a difficult position. Transformational leaders are able to communicate their vision to the staff, at the same time identify the constraints within their role.
2. ***Inspirational motivation***: The leader must be able to encourage others to achieve organizational goals and aspirations, while also achieving his or her own. Motivation is absolutely necessary. Does staff sit on committees in which major decisions are made? Does the organization have shared governance? Is it truly practiced? Becoming inspirational is far more difficult because many nurses develop leadership skills on the traditional managerial basis. Inspiration flows downward like a cascade—therefore it is something a new leader must exhibit.
3. ***Intellectual stimulation:*** Using evidence-based practice approaches is a way to empower staff to approach problems. Technologic and literary facilities should be available for all staff to use. This will reinforce the need for continuing education instead of relying on "this is how I always did it or how I learned it." Although organizations have encouraged staff to continue their education, formally and informally, no one has ever encouraged them to "share" their knowledge with others. A transformational leader will encourage staff to share articles and knowledge learned with others through formal and informal dissemination methods.
4. ***Individualized consideration:*** A true leader must be supportive. Leaders have a responsibility to care for their staff. Regular positive feedback, staff appraisals, peer reviews, and 360° evaluations are just some examples of how to increase a person's value and self-esteem, thereby increasing performance. Empowerment has long been linked to self-efficacy: when one increases, so does the other. Does staff feel part of a team; is their voice heard in meetings? Does staff feel stifled from the hierarchy?

Let us contrast transactional theory and transformational theory to that of Abraham Maslow. Maslow's hierarchy of needs theory is based on a pyramid. At the bottom of the pyramid are our basic needs; the second level is security; the third level is relationship; the fourth level is self-esteem; and the fifth level is self-actualization. Transactional leadership reaches the second level of Maslow's pyramid, whereas transformational leadership reaches the fifth level of Maslow's pyramid.

CONTEMPORARY LEADERS OF OUR TIME

One of the most contemporary leaders of our time is Dr. Stephen Covey. Dr. Covey's theory is principle-centered leadership. Dr. Covey wrote a best-selling book titled *The 7 Habits of Highly Effective People*. The 7 principles outlined in this book are as follows:

1. Be proactive.
2. Begin with the end in mind.
3. Put first things first.
4. Think win/win.
5. Seek first to understand, then to be understood.
6. Synergize.
7. Sharpen the saw.

The 7 principles are rather self-explanatory. Let us review 2 in detail. One of the most important principles is that of seeking first to understand, then to be understood. What Dr. Covey is referring to here is the art of communication. Often, we will respond quickly before having really understood the message that has been sent. Dr. Covey states that we should clarify the message before responding. He states that if the message was clear and understood, our response would be appropriate, and human interaction would be much more beneficial.

The other principle is sharpening the saw. By this, Dr. Covey implies that we should consistently practice the first 6 principles so that we can perfect them. When one thinks about it, although these principles are often used in management and leadership circles, they really are great principles for everyday life.

The next leader to be discussed is Dr. Peter Senge. Dr. Senge wrote the book titled *The Fifth Discipline*. In this book, he describes how organizations have to be in a constant learning mode. This can be done through many venues of education. He also states that human beings will create webs of significance and work across disciplines to achieve the goals of the organization. He states that management's role is to allow this to occur. Many times managers are taught that when people work together they are doing something evil, and the role of the manager is to cut down the grapevine. Dr. Senge takes the opposite view—that most times when people are working together, they are doing something good for the organization.

Another leader is Dr. Tom Peters. Dr. Peters' leadership style is nontraditional. For example, he states that the title of the CEO should be CDO, that is, chief destruction officer. He states that the CDO or the CEO should always be looking at things to tear down and rebuild where necessary. He also states that if an employee cannot say how he or she contributed to the workplace that day, he or she does not belong there. All employees have to embrace the mission of the organization and make it successful.

Another leader, Marcus Buckingham, worked for the Gallup poll for several years and developed a very simplistic theory. This theory is based on employees doing what they do best. This theory infers that an organization should structure jobs so that the worker is doing everything that he or she is educated to do and what he or she likes to do best. Should jobs be structured in this way, employees will continue to want to work at that company and will continually improve their performance.

OTHER THEORIES

Systems Theory

There are 2 major types of systems: open and closed. All systems involve 3 major concepts: input, process/throughput, and output. The difference between an open system and a closed system is that an open system interacts with its environment, whereas a closed system does not. A computer system is an excellent example of a closed environment. There is input into the hard drive. There is throughput as items are processed on the hard drive. There is output in the form of a presentation that is viewable on a screen or a printout. Other than data input, there is no interaction with the environment. Anyone who has seasonal allergies understands the concept of interaction with an environment. Take health care organizations as an example. There is certainly interaction with the environment. The following lists some of the environments with which health care organizations interact:

- Regulators, i.e., State Department of Health
- Accreditors, i.e., Joint Commission or Det Norske Veritas Healthcare, Inc. (DNV-HC)
- Payers, insurance payment, self-pay
- Vendors, suppliers of items that we use in health care
- Can you think of any others?

Systems Theory and Framework

A **system** consists of a set of interrelated and interdependent, coordinated components designed to meet common goals. Ludwig von Bertalanffy emphasized that systems are open to and interact with their environments. They acquire new properties and continually evolve. Rather than reducing the overall entity to the properties of its parts, systems theory focuses on how the parts are arranged and interact with each other to create a "whole." Systems theory has now been incorporated into every facet of life, from family systems to information systems, banking systems, and, of course, health care systems.

Basic Principles of a Systems Approach

- A system is greater than the sum of its parts. It requires investigation of the whole situation rather than 1 or 2 aspects of a problem. Mistakes cannot be blamed on one person; rather a systems analyst would investigate how the mistake occurred within a subsystem and look for opportunities to make corrections in the processes used.
- The portion of the world studied (system) must exhibit some predictability.
- Although each subsystem is a self-contained unit, it is part of a wider and higher order.
- The central objective of a system can be identified by the fact that other objectives will be sacrificed to attain the central objective.
- Every system, living or mechanical, is an information system. One must analyze how suitable the symbols used are for information transmission.
- An open system and its environment are highly interrelated.
- A highly complex system may have to be broken into subsystems, so each can be analyzed and understood before being reassembled into a whole.
- A system consists of a set of objectives and their relationships.
- A system is a dynamic network of interconnecting elements. A change in only one of the elements must produce change in all the others.
- When subsystems are arranged in a series, the output of one is the input for another; therefore, process alterations in one require alterations in other subsystems.
- All systems tend toward equilibrium, which is a balance of various forces within and outside of a system.
- The boundary of a system can be redrawn at will by a system analyst.
- To be viable, a system must be strongly goal directed, governed by feedback, and have the ability to adapt to changing circumstances.

Taking the definitions listed here, look at the following example of how systems theory works:

> *You want to set your home thermostat. How does that thermostat work? When the temperature falls, the thermostat tells the heater to turn on. Heat is then generated from the furnace or heater. When you reach the ideal temperature, the thermostat tells the heater to turn off. Now look at it from a systems theory viewpoint.*

Input—The gas or electricity, which comes from the power company

Output—Heat

Throughput—The thermostat monitors the temperature; the thermostat sends a signal to the heater to turn on; the thermostat sends a signal to the heater to turn off; the gas is burned; and the fan turns on and blows warm air into the room.

Feedback—When the temperature falls below the desired level, the thermostat sends a signal to the heater. When the temperature reaches the desired level, the thermostat sends a signal to the heater to turn off.

The U.S. health care system contains various components of health services delivery, which are loosely coordinated. Human resources consist of the various types and categories of workers engaged in delivering health care (e.g., physicians, nurses, dentists, pharmacists, other doctoral trained professionals, and allied health professionals) along with ancillary workers, such as those in billing, marketing, and public relations. These resources are intertwined with health care access. Look at rural areas: Health care may be restricted owing to lack of health care providers, lack of financing for health care, and lack of technology available.

System resources influence the development of and change in physical infrastructure (such as hospitals, nursing homes, and clinics). Most services are delivered via outpatient care rather than through inpatient institutions. System outcomes are the critical issues and concerns surrounding the health services system that can be accomplished. What is its primary objective? Are the health services cost-effective? Did the care meet the quality standards? Access, cost, and quality are the main outcome criteria used to evaluate success of a health care delivery system. System outlook is how the dynamic health care system is looking. Is it forward looking?

The clinical and administrative processes in today's health care environment are increasingly complex. A complex system is characterized by a connected network of various entities from which a higher order emerges. This requires the organization to **ADAPT to CHANGE**. To do this, it is important to look at health care organizations (single organization or multiorganization) as living complex adaptive systems rather than as traditional "dead" systems.

A chapter on systems thinking is also included in this book.

Chaos Theory

Chaos theory was developed in the mid-1980s by a researcher/physicist at the Massachusetts Institute of Technology. In the science of physics, every belief up to the development of this theory stated that things do not happen randomly or chaotically; everything is predictable. An example of this would be an infant's crib mobile. A mobile can have both small arms and large arms, and, depending on the weight of each arm, the mobile can be perfectly balanced; again this is predictable. What about Isaac Newton's law of gravity? When one throws the ball up into the air, it comes down because of gravitational pull. Again, this is predictable.

Chaos theory developed from studying computers. The computer uses binary code. The researcher predicted that if he programmed the computer with a whole number, such as the number 2, and instructed the computer to run this number 500 times, it would graph a straight line. That is exactly what happened. Then the researcher programmed the computer to run a fraction of the number 2, for example, 2.002. Again he predicted that the computer would graph a straight line. To his surprise, the computer did not graph a straight line. The researcher discovered what he called a butterfly effect, in which the graph went off the line and then came back down onto the line. He then started to believe that physics may not be so predictable; that is, things do happen randomly and chaotically. He started to think about the human sciences: how can anything be predictable? We know that medicine and nursing are not predictable sciences.

Chaos theory is a mathematical discipline that studies the functioning of complex systems. Originally used to predict weather variations, some of its concepts can be adapted onto other areas, such as health care. Remember that complex systems are always in motion. They run through some type of cycle but always try to create some kind of equilibrium, not duplicating situations. Within chaos theory, there is a lack of order within the system, although the system obeys its own rules and regulations. It is dynamically unstable, therefore unpredictable. There are 2 main components of chaos theory:

- Systems (no matter how complex) rely on an underlying order.
- Small or simple systems and events can cause complex behaviors and events.

Therefore, any slight change in the initial conditions makes predicting future or past outcomes impossible. Tom Peters in 1988 wrote a book titled *Thriving on Chaos*. In this book, he stated that organizations that will be successful must be flexible and adapt to changing business environment. Those organizations that do not adapt and that are not flexible will not survive. Have we not seen numerous hospital closures over the past several years? Those are the hospitals and health care systems that could not adapt to a changing environment.

Complexity Theory

Complexity theory grew from chaos theory. It states that the world is very complex and chaotic. This certainly describes health care and nursing today. The key is that as leaders we need to be flexible and able to adapt to a constantly changing environment, changing norms, and changing political forces.

Complex Adaptive Systems Theory or Complexity Theory

Complex adaptive systems theory (complexity theory) is composed of concepts that seek to explain complex phenomenon using different methodologies. It combines chaos theory, psychology, computer science, systems theory, and fuzzy logic to deal with systems as they are and not by breaking them down into their parts. It attempts to tell how systems create their own order, pattern, and structure. The underlying premise is that there is a hidden order to behavior within a complex system. Managers learn that these systems, if allowed to function on their own, bring about their own order. The employees behave as a single unit and respond to the changes within their environment. Complex systems will go to the "edge of chaos" but never fall over that edge. There is enough creativity, ideas, and strength to sustain life.

These 3 theories all form the basis for nursing leaders to develop new strategies in times of chaos, complexity, and change. Leaders must recognize when chaos works (great ideas can come from those times) and when structure works (as in specific procedures or technology). Unfortunately, our present-day health care organizations are built on traditional concepts, and often management does not adapt to the need for change and growth. Dee Hock, in his 2005 book *One From Many*, describes the development of a chaotic organization, where "the behavior of any self-organizing and self-governing organization harmoniously blends characteristics of chaos and order" (p. 13). By recognizing and understanding these theories, a leader can determine trends, support change, and expand the unit or organization to sustain its identity, purpose, and overall focus, yielding better overall outcomes.

Systems Thinking

Based on the information provided earlier, a nursing leader needs to adapt to systems thinking. This holistic approach looks at the system as a whole and how its interrelated parts function within the larger organization. This means that the effective leader balances creativity and ideas with practicality. However, no matter what, the leader must deal with change. Continual change is the reality of health care. Not only will the nursing leader need to adapt to change, but he or she will also need to support (not always manage) others in changing. This is a journey that must be taken together with those with whom you work. The leader must also note that there will be resistance to change and that taking time to listen is the better course of action than bulldozing ahead.

Change Theory

Change is inherent in the world that we live in today. For organizations to survive, they must be willing to change and adapt to what is going on in their environment. One of the most noted theorists on change is Kurt Lewin, who defined 3 stages of change.

Unfreezing—This is where the organization senses a need for change, for example, pressures from the government and payers to move to an electronic health record. In the unfreezing stage, it is important to make others aware of the need for change and to ascertain their thoughts about the change. It is also critical to start to identify change agents, who agree with the change and are willing to engage others in making the change.

Movement—This is where the plan is developed. Goals and objectives are formulated. A timeline is developed for implementation of the change. It is critical in this stage to identify those who support the change and, more important, those who are resistors of the change. The goal is to get the resistors to recognize and understand the need for change. It is also vital for management to be present and available on every shift to provide support to staff as the change is implemented.

Refreezing—This is when the change becomes a permanent part of the organization. The change should be evaluated and revised if necessary. One can learn a lot once implementation occurs, because at times during the planning process, certain things cannot be seen or ascertained. It is also critical for management to be available on every shift at this phase to make the change a permanent part of the organization.

CASE EXAMPLE

A hospital for whom I consulted had implemented a new care delivery model on an oncology unit. There had not been a lot of education done to educate the staff about this change. The oncology unit had three 12-bed modules. The CEO and the chief nursing officer (CNO) had decided to implement the new nursing care delivery model on 1 of the 12-bed modules. The nursing care delivery model was team based. There was 1 registered nurse (RN) assigned to every 6 patients; thus there were 2 RNs assigned to this module. There was 1 patient care technician assigned to all 12 patients. There was 1 manager assigned to the 12 patients. My role was to develop an education program for the staff. This was done, and when the program was presented, I learned that the model was not working up to the expectations of the staff. The problem was that 1 patient care technician could not care for 12 oncology patients. The staff recommended that having 2 patient care technicians would correct the problem. This was discussed with the nurse manager, and an additional patient care technician was added to the model. Once this was accomplished, the staff really valued this new nursing care delivery model, and it was soon able to be implemented on other nursing units in the hospital. This case study demonstrates the importance of evaluation and listening to staff, as they are closest to the product of care delivery.

Emotional Intelligence

What Exactly Is Emotional Intelligence?

Emotional intelligence is the ability to monitor and, more important, develop strategies to deal with one's emotions. It is people, emotions, and behavior management. This is not new and actually began with Thorndike in the 1920s. Goleman in the 1990s explained the differences between emotional intelligence (EQ) and the intelligence quotient (IQ). Salovey and Mayer (1990) are also gurus in the field. According to Salovey and Mayer (1990), EQ is the ability to monitor one's own and others' feelings and emotions, to discriminate among them, and to use this information to guide one's thinking and actions.

For years it was thought that the best leaders were those who had a very high IQs. It makes some sense that the most brilliant individuals would make the best leaders. Research over the years has demonstrated the opposite, however; that is, the most successful leaders are the ones who have a higher EQ compared with IQ. An emotionally intelligent leader is one who can connect to people, and the organizations that connect to people are the most successful.

There are different models for EQ. The key is for one to be able to identify an individual's emotions, understand those emotions, and, most important, utilize those emotions by connecting to the other person.

Appreciative Inquiry

As a CNO, I always focused on problems, until one day my critical care director said to me, "Do you consider that most of the time, things go right? We have over 12,000 admissions each year and a lot of things go right." This was great learning for me and is what appreciative inquiry is all about. This theory emphasizes what an organization does best and then takes that to a higher level. For example, a hospital may have a cardiac catheterization laboratory that performs interventions, but the closest hospital for open heart surgery is more than 60 miles away. The first hospital then develops a strategic plan to bring open heart surgery to its region. The certificate of need is approved. The first hospital then implements a heart surgery program and also adds an electrophysiology laboratory to their services. After a couple of years with this program running, they see that they have very good outcomes. Then they decide to go further and aim to be the best hospital for cardiac outcomes in their state.

Types of Businesses

Sole proprietor	The owner is the business.
Partnerships	Two or more individuals form a business. Partnerships can be general or limited. In a general partnership, the partners share equally. An example of a limited partner would be an investor in the business.
Corporation	This is when a business incorporates in the state where the business is located. Articles of incorporation are filed. Bylaws are developed. By incorporating, individuals are more protected from lawsuits. A corporation is invisible. It is not the offices on Main Street. It is paperwork filed with a state.

Concept of piercing the corporate veil. When incorporated insurance is taken to cover employees of the corporation, a veil is created, so to speak, that protects individuals. This veil can be pierced if an individual commits an act of negligence such as malpractice. In situations like this the insurance company will target the individual rather than the corporation.

Board of Trustees (Governors)

Corporations are governed by a Board of Trustees/Governors. The governing body has a fiduciary responsibility. Board members must be honest and ethical and avoid conflicts of interest. The bylaws of the organization will define titles of officers, when meetings are conducted, and how board members are notified of meetings. Board members' role is oversight and not day-to-day operational. Their role is to provide a different view and perspective and to question why certain processes are done in the manner that they are accomplished. This role is to assure the sustainability and financial success of the organization and to meet the needs of the community that the organization serves. One of the primary focuses of board members today is on the quality of care that is provided. Usually the CEO is a voting board member. Other members of the executive staff members usually attend meetings as invited guests. Some organizations appoint the CNO/Chief Nurse Executive (CNE) as a voting board member. The American Academy of Nursing has a goal to get 10,000 nurses appointed to boards.

Hospital boards must assure that a Community Health Needs Assessment is conducted every 3 years. This is one of the mandates in the Patient Protection and Affordable Care Act (ACA, 2010). A hospital must complete a Community Health Needs Assessment at least every 3 years. Input is obtained from the broader community. It is important to include public health experts in this process. Hospitals must describe how community health needs are addressed as well as identify any needs not being addressed and provide an explanation as to why these health needs are not being addressed.

Hospitals must also provide an annual report to the community on the services provided as well as key financial performance, for example, the dollars expended on charity care annually. The American Hospital Association has sample forms available for this purpose. In a health network with multiple hospitals, a report to each hospital community must be provided. The meeting date and time are scheduled and announced to the community. A certain number of board members as well as the CEO and other executive staff members must be present at the meeting. Attendance is documented. Should no one show up to the meeting from the community, board members and staff wait for around 15 minutes and document that no one from the community attended the meeting.

Management Process

The following defines the 5 functions of managers (Fayol, 1949):

1. Planning
    a. Strategic
    b. Tactical
2. Organizing
3. Coordinating
4. Directing
5. Controlling

The Work of Management

The following defines the work of management:

1. Allocating resources
2. Handling exceptions
3. Disseminating information

4. Resolving conflicts
5. Solving problems
6. Managing workers

Important Managerial Skills

The following defines the skill set of management (Mintzberg, 1975):

1. Developing peer relationships
2. Carrying out negotiations
3. Motivating subordinates
4. Resolving conflicts
5. Establishing information networks and disseminating information
6. Making decisions in conditions of extreme ambiguity
7. Allocating resources

Eight Practices of Effective Executives (Drucker, 2004)

1. What needs to be done?
2. What is right for the enterprise?
3. They developed action plans.
4. They took responsibility for decisions.
5. They took responsibility for communicating.
6. They were focused on opportunities, not problems.
7. They ran productive meetings.
8. They thought and said "we" not "I."

The Mind-Set of Management (Gosling and Mintzberg, 2003)

1. Reflective mind-set: managing self
2. Analytic mind-set: managing organizations
3. Worldly mind-set: managing context
4. Collaborative mind-set: managing relationships
5. Action mind-set: managing change

Leadership Responsibilities

With regard to leadership, nurse executives are responsible for many key areas. These are inclusive of the following:

- Client care management
- Managing clinical nursing practice

Operational Management

- Managing fiscal and material resources
- Complying with regulatory and professional standards

- Participating in strategic planning for the organization
- Developing a strategic plan for the nursing division

Human Resources Management

- Developing personnel
- Fostering interdisciplinary and collaborative relationships
- Hiring employees
- Disciplining employees
- Firing employees when necessary

A snapshot of nursing management

Patient Care Responsibilities

- Client care management
- Managing clinical nursing practice

Operational Management

- Managing fiscal and material resources
- Complying with regulatory and professional standards
- Participating in strategic planning

Human Resource Management

- Developing personnel
- Fostering interdisciplinary and collaborative relationships

Client Care Management and Clinical Nursing Practice

Nursing has evolved over the years. Nursing services have organized care under various delivery models. These models will be discussed here, as at times, for various reasons, older models of nursing care get reused. For example, nursing services may want to implement primary care with an all-RN staff, yet constraints will not permit this; therefore another type of model is used.

Functional Nursing

This is a task-oriented model of nursing care delivery. Each nurse is responsible for specific tasks. For example, there is a medication nurse whose main responsibility is the administration of medications and taking new medication orders. Depending on the practice environment, many nurses get disillusioned with this model, as a nurse is much more than just a medicine nurse. Because nursing services are in multiple environments today, some nursing services use this model. For example, a methadone maintenance clinic usually has a nurse whose sole responsibility is the administration of methadone to a set number of patients at a set time each day.

Team Nursing

Team nursing generally uses an RN as the team leader, and other types of nursing staff make up the team, for example, a licensed practical or vocational nurse and a nursing assistant or technician. The team is assigned to a set group of patients. The team works together to achieve good patient outcomes. This model once was used in acute care hospitals; however, this model now tends to work well in rehabilitation environments; for example, in addiction treatment centers, many licensed practical or vocational nurses and residential service technicians are used in the care model.

Modular Nursing

Over the years, team nursing evolved to modular nursing. The main intent of modular nursing was to put the nursing team closest to the patient. Some hospitals relocated the nursing station to where the team was located. Should 3 teams be on a specific unit, then there would be 3 decentralized nursing stations.

Primary Care

Depending on the literature that one reads, many consider Dr. Joyce Clifford, who was the CNE at Boston Beth Israel Medical Center for several years, the mother of primary care. Others consider Marie Manthey from Minnesota as the mother of primary care. Suffice it to say that Dr. Clifford was extremely successful back in the early 1970s with the care delivery model. Boston Beth Israel Medical Center, under Dr. Clifford's leadership, was rated several times as one of the best places for women to work. The pure primary care model was an all-RN staff. The RN was accountable for patient care 24/7 and would map out the plan of care. I had the opportunity to work in a new hospital back in 1975. The hospital had 110 adult patient beds. The physical design of the hospital was in the shape of a "Y," with 18 patients in each arm of the "Y" and the nurses' station in the center of the "Y." Private rooms, where the most critical patients were placed, were closest to the nurses' station. The first floor was the medical floor and the second was the surgical floor. The CNE of this organization was also very innovative in this model of care. She had the foresight to have dietary distribute water pitchers and dinner trays collected. Unit secretaries were educated to transcribe all orders inclusive of medication orders. Nurses had to verify and sign off on these. The CNE basically attempted to keep the nurse at the bedside with the patient and at the same time reduce the indirect care that nurses always have provided, i.e., managing water pitchers and dinner trays. Many hospitals attempted to implement this pure primary care model in their organizations; however, usually RN staffing shortages or finances prohibited it in many places.

Modified Primary Care

As many hospitals could not employ an all-RN staff and as some tasks do not need to be completed by an RN, hospitals then moved to a modified primary care model. This model incorporated the addition of patient care technicians, whereby a patient care technician or nursing assistant would be paired with the RN. Many of these individuals were in nursing school or contemplating attending a nursing program. They were educated to do intake and output measurements, empty Foley catheters, do finger-stick blood glucose tests, take vital signs, do bed baths, feed patients who required such, and do other tasks within their scope of practice.

This model of care was in place for some time in many hospitals and still exists in some organizations to this day.

Patient-Focused Care

In the early 1990s a few statisticians analyzed hospitals as to where the dollars were spent and where inefficiencies existed. For example, postoperative patients with total hip replacement would have an X-ray on postoperative day 1. These patients would have to be transported to the radiology department, which involved an attendant's time and associated costs. A new model of care emerged that focused more on the patient. Why not group like patients together on the same nursing unit? Rather than transporting patients to the necessary service, why not bring the service to the patient? Two new terms were coined for this model. One was *concentric ring*, which simply meant to group like patients together. In this example, put all patients with total joint procedures on the same unit. Then if an X-ray is required on postoperative day 1, place a satellite X-ray room on the unit itself. To achieve this effectively, the nursing unit had to have some physical space changes made. The second term was that the design of the unit had to be *fungible*, which simply means flexible. What happens when total joint procedures become same-day surgical procedures and the inpatient unit is no longer required? If the design of the unit is fungible, the satellite X-ray room can easily be converted to a satellite pharmacy for the admixture of various drugs and intravenous (IV) fluids, as now the unit is a post–intensive care unit. If a hospital was wise, they would analyze the cost of implementation of such a model. Many concluded that it was no more cost-effective than other models. Some borrowed ideas from focused care and implemented them into their other nursing model, oftentimes that being a modified primary care model.

Relationship-Based Care

Marie Manthey is most noted for this model of care. It does make a lot of sense in that a nurse has relationships with patients and other staff. This model incorporates concepts of caring, not only caring for the patient but also caring for each other. Such a model may incorporate a therapeutic room on the nursing unit where staff can go to decompress and relieve stress. Running water, lounge chairs, soft music, and other environmental factors to relieve stress may be part of the environment. Manthey's newest model merges primary care with relationship-based care.

Family-Centered Care

This model recognizes the importance of family. For the sake of this book, family refers to any person or persons who are important to the patient. It may be a biological family member, a significant other, or a friend. On another note, what about a patient's pets? The key is that the family is incorporated as an important part of the care model. Pediatrics was the first to initiate this—the permitting of parents to remain with the child overnight. We now see this being incorporated into adult nursing units and critical care units. It has been recognized how important family members contribute to a loved one's well-being.

Case Example 1

When our grandson was admitted with a rotavirus infection at 7 years of age, we were permitted to be with him through procedures as well as sleep in his room. We knew that this contributed to his recovery. We had raised our grandson from birth, so, to him, we were his parents and he had never been separated from us.

Case Example 2

An operative experience can be frightening for any child. A CNO at an acute care hospital had hired a pediatric Clinical Nurse Specialist and a Child Life Specialist. These individuals created a unique environment for children having surgery. A preoperative holding room was decorated with a children's motif. Parents could stay with the child in the holding room. There were objects and videotapes for children to play with. The child would then be sedated with nasal midazolam (Versed) rather than an injection. As the child would be sleepy, the lights were dimmed and soft music was played. The child then would be transported with or carried by his parents right into the operating room, which was decorated the same as the preoperative holding room. After the child was asleep, the parents then waited in the patient waiting room. When the surgery was completed and the child transferred to the postanesthesia care unit, the parents were waiting by the child's bedside. This service created very satisfied customers. In addition, physicians who were working in more than one hospital started to send all of their pediatric surgeries to this hospital, as the parents raved about the service.

The Synergy Model of Patient Care

This model was developed by the American Association of Critical Care Nurses. The model focuses on moving the patient through the system safely and with expert nursing care. The competencies of the nurse are aligned with the needs of the patient. This is something that nursing has tried to do for years, and now, as a model, it validates that this is one way to assure quality patient care.

Other Perspectives on Models of Nursing Care Delivery

One thing that many nursing executives have learned is that there is no one model for each type of nursing unit. The vast majority of nurses want things standardized. For example, if primary care is the model, then that model must exist for each nursing unit. The reality is that every nursing unit has its own culture. Patient's needs vary from unit to unit. It makes sense then that what should really be in place in most organizations is an eclectic model whereby a different model is in place on different units based on the needs of the patient and the staff. A key part is to have the nursing staff on each unit define what model works best for them, as they are the ones who ultimately will make the model succeed or fail.

Case Management

Dr. Karen Zander is one of the leaders in the case management nursing model. The belief is that educated nurses should do case management by their specialty, not necessarily by patient geographic region. For example, if a nurse's specialty is caring for patients with cerebral vascular accident (CVA), then the case manager nurse should care for patients with CVA regardless of geographic location. Zander was focused on quality care to patients. The belief was that the case manager should manage the patient prehospital, intrahospital, and posthospital discharge. The goal was to keep the patient well and out of the hospital. Part of Zander's model was the creation of the critical pathway. The critical pathway defined what should occur on each day of a patient's hospital stay based on the diagnosis. Variations in care had to be explained. For example, a patient with total knee replacement was placed on a 3-day pathway. On day 1 after the surgical procedure, the patient's IV line should be removed. By day 3 the patient should be discharged. On postoperative day 2, if the IV line was still in place, was this secondary to a patient problem (the patient had continuous vomiting requiring IV fluids) or was it a system problem (the physician forgot to write an order to remove the IV line)? Managed care companies have picked up on Zander's work and have concluded that, if every patient in a U.S. hospital was on a critical pathway, there would be thousands of patient-days saved, which translates to the reduction of thousands of dollars of care. Because the risk for infection in any inpatient health care environment is high, it makes perfect sense to get the patient to transgress the systems as safely and efficiently as possible. Is it not interesting today that the Center for Medicare and Medicaid Services is focused on efficiency in hospitals?

Strategic Management

Strategic management and planning really has its roots in the certificate-of-need process that states had to undergo to add or build new services. Every 5 years a long-range plan had to be revisited and updated for a state to participate in the certificate-of-need process. Earlier there were health system agencies that plan services geographically. When managed care became a reality as a reimbursement methodology, strategic planning became vital to the organization survival. All of a sudden the long-range plan had to become a strategic plan, which is a living document that gets reviewed and updated periodically.

Strategic management is a process by which leaders set goals and objectives for the organization, determine the resources needed to achieve them, and establish policies and procedures for acquiring and using those resources.

Strategic management includes a community needs assessment, which should drive a strategic plan for the respective organization. This can be done by strategic planning, which includes a **SWOT** analysis

S = the organization's strengths
W = the organization's weakness
O = the organization's opportunities
T = the organization's threats

The higher in the organization's chain of command, the greater the portion of time that the leader or manager will spend on strategic planning. Strengths and weaknesses are internal components. These are related to resources, programs, and operations in key areas of the organization, such as operations, management, products, and finances. The external components are the opportunities and threats. These involve the industry, the marketplace, the economy, the political climate, technology, competition, and strategic partnerships. Some organizations include a **PEST** analysis. **PEST** stands for

P = Political environment
E = Economic environment
S = Sociocultural environment
T = Technologic environment

A **PEST** analysis looks at a much broader picture. For example, looking at the political environment, what effect can a presidential or gubernatorial election have on a state or country? This depends on which candidate gets voted into office. The strategic planner is the advisor or a facilitator to line management decision makers. The program executive is the key strategist but not the strategic planner. Strategic planning is not an isolated process. It is integrated with other functions in the program management process.

Changes in reimbursement methodologies and the pressure on cost containment have shaped the strategic focus in many health care organizations today.

Nurse executives and unit-level managers are essential to the strategic planning process. The current challenge is to identify ways in which to provide value through the provision of quality care that are also cost-effective.

Strategic planning asks a few questions.

1. Where are we currently?
2. Where do we need to go?
3. How do we get there?

The primary purpose of strategic planning is to provide for the organization's growth and development. It involves an intense environmental analysis, both internal and external. It involves the development of goals and strategy. It can provide a unified vision and goals for the organization to accomplish. It also can help ensure that the necessary resources are available to carry out strategic initiatives. It defines what will be done to achieve the outcomes.

Steps in the Strategic Planning Process

Develop a strategic vision and mission

- Identify and include partnership opportunities in the community and the business world.
- Key stakeholders are crucial for success.
- Set objectives.
- Develop strategies to achieve the objectives.
- Implement the strategies.
- Evaluate the outcomes.

The strategic planning process will identify the following:

- Strategic issues
- Stragetic initiatives—what the organization is willing to take on
- A business plan and a timeline for implementation of the strategic initiatives

Some Other Thoughts on Strategic Management and Planning

Organizational strategy must be responsive to the environment. What changes the environment? Examples are demographic shifts, sociocultural changes, and technology.

An example of strategic planning that most organizations are embarking on is the elderly population. When we look at data, individuals aged 65+ and 85+ years are some of the fastest-growing populations in the United States. As many elderly are being cared for in hospitals today, different strategies have been used. An example of one hospital's strategic initiative to care better for the elderly as well as increase patient volume and revenue is the development of an area of the emergency department that focuses on geriatric care, i.e., the geriatric emergency department. An entire chapter on strategic planning is also included in this book.

Strategic Partnerships

For any business to survive the turbulent health care milieu today, it is necessary that organizations establish partnerships with like and other businesses. The goal of such partnerships or alliances would be for the mutual benefit of each organization. The following provides some examples.

Example 1. A community hospital system that provides cardiac catheterization services aligns with a university hospital for advanced cardiac services that the community hospital system does not provide, for example, open heart surgery, transcatheter aortic valve replacement, and advanced laboratory services. This same community hospital system may align with a university hospital for cancer treatment services, as the university hospital would have research treatment protocols.

Example 2. A hospital system aligns with a university that has a medical school, a nursing school, and a school of public health. The hospital system decides to build a new hospital on ground near the university. Both the hospital and the university will benefit from shared resources, such as dietary and environmental services. Both the hospital and the university further benefit, as students in the university's programs can obtain clinical experiences at the hospital system.

Example 3. A hospital system aligns with a university for the sharing of faculty from the university. For example, a nurse researcher works 1 day per week at the hospital, directing the nursing research program at the hospital. The hospital benefits from increased research activity as well as the achievement of Magnet status.

Communication

Communication is a critical aspect of any organization. One can compare communication with blood circulation in the human body. Just as blood carries hemoglobin molecules to keep us alive and nourish us, communication is the critical aspect of keeping an organization functioning at peak performance. Deprived of oxygen, cells will malfunction and die. Deprived of necessary information, individuals and departments within organizations cannot function. Research evidence suggests that accurate, relevant information and appropriate quantities improve decision making and other kinds of performance for individuals and groups.

Let us examine familiar managerial roles. These roles are inclusive of planning, leading, directing, organizing, and controlling. Managers will function in various roles. These roles include formal authority; interpersonal roles, such as figurehead, leader, and liaison; information roles, such as monitor, disseminator, and spokesperson; and decision roles, such as entrepreneur, intrapreneur, disturbance handler, resource allocator, and negotiator. Let us break down each one of these roles.

Formal Authority

A manager's position is endowed with status and authority by the organization. The position is critical to a network of interpersonal relationships that lead to inputs and outputs.

Interpersonal Roles

A figurehead is a symbolic position, for example, one who presents awards or entertains visitors. The leader is to accomplish the task and goals of the organization. Much of this role centers on the leader functioning as a liaison and communicator.

Information Roles

In this role the leader is to monitor and obtain information on operations. The leader will disseminate information to those affected. A spokesperson will represent his or her unit.

Decision Roles

A leader who is an entrepreneur is innovative and creative outside the organization. A leader who is an intrapreneur is innovative and creative within the organization. Decision roles also require the leader to be a disturbance handler whereby the leader will handle controversy. The leader also is a resource allocator in this role. The leader parcels out limited time, money, materials, and talent. The leader also has to function as a negotiator dealing with on-the-spot bargaining and exchanging.

What prevails in each of these preceding roles that were discussed is the concept of communication. Many studies document that managers spend the vast amount of their time communicating with others.

There are 3 major types or categories of communication: up the organization, down the organization, and across the organization. Upward communication is information that gets carried upward as the work progresses and news of problems for decision making comes from the subordinate or the employee to the manager. This information is often filtered. Downward communication flows down the organization to inform, direct, and control. This information also may be filtered. The communication comes from the manager down to the employee or the subordinate. Lateral communication, what we call diagonal communication, occurs between multiple departments. This form of communication is primarily used for coordination and problem-solving. It is the most complex form of communication and involves a great deal of time. This type of communication is challenging because it involves intergroup relationships, it is irregular, it can interfere with daily routines, the numbers to manage can be great, it mushrooms and increases in quantity quickly, required relationships are often ambiguous, and management sometimes keeps adding a new specialist to the equation.

Networks of communication are less unstable and a significant element in the art of managing is knowingly shifts and importance of information in acquiring, sharing, and making effective decisional use of the information.

The Communication Process

There are 6 major components to the communication process: thinking, encoding, transmitting the signal, perceiving, decoding, and understanding. Let us take a look at each one of these separately.

Thinking. Here the person who wants to communicate something has the genesis of the idea and frames that idea or message in the sender's mind.

Encoding. Here the communicator places the thought into some form of possible communication. There are multiple forms of communication today, such as verbal communication and multiple forms of electronic communication.

Transmitting the Signal. Here the actual message is broadcast via some medium. The next 3 forms of communication involve the one receiving the message.

Perceiving. The receiver must perceive the incoming communication with one or more senses, such as sight, hearing, feeling, taste, and smell.

Decoding. The receiver puts the incoming communication into some form that will make it understandable.

Understanding. The receiver understands the message hopefully as it was intended to be understood by the sender. Understanding involves thought transmission. One can see that, even though the 6 forms of communication sound simplistic, anything can go wrong with any one step and the message will probably not be transmitted or perceived correctly. Let us review a case study. Haney (1979, p. 318) describes an event that occurred in Kemble, England. Four Royal Air Force jets speeding across England, Tuesday when the rear pilot radioed: quote you are on fire-eject. Flight Lieut. John Rust, aged 30 years, bailed out of one plane. Flight Lieut. Richard Duckett, aged 27 years, bailed out of another plane. Rust's plane was on fire. Both pilots landed uninjured. What was wrong with that communication? It is obvious that the message was not clear. The person radioing these pilots should have stated which pilot's plane was on fire. This was a costly event; 2 Royal Air Force jets are not inexpensive. These jets had to land somewhere, and hopefully they landed over the ocean and not into a town, which could have caused further damage as well as the loss of life. In summary of this case study, our communication must be direct and clear and must state all the key facts (Haney, 1979 as cited in Umiker, 1979).

Barriers to Understanding. Another way that messages may be perceived incorrectly is the barriers to understanding. These include lack of congruence, distorted perceptions, distorted source, defensive behavior, and distortions from the past.

It is important for the leader to create a good communication climate. The following are some examples of creating that climate.

Defensive	versus	Supportive
Evaluation	versus	Description
Control	versus	Being problem-oriented
Strategy	versus	Spontaneity
Neutrality	versus	Empathy
Superiority	versus	Equality
Certainty	versus	Provisionalism

Other Thoughts on Communication

Communication must be honest. The leader must create an environment of trustworthiness and credibility. Transparency equates to honesty. Our leaders are honest individuals who will do almost anything for the organization.

According to Peter Senge, organizations are learning institutions. Informal groups of people perform the work. Managers are not always in the loop or aware. Oftentimes, informal groups cannot be identified. Management's role should allow this to happen, unless the communication is dysfunctional.

Communication also involves conflict. Conflict is defined as a state of disharmony. It is important to recognize that legitimate differences do exist. There may be disagreement on goals or priorities, on facts of the particular case or situation, on interpretation of the facts, or on resource allocation. And individuals also may lack values clarification. The positive aspect of conflict management is that it can bring about change. Conflict management can also develop creativity, clarify issues, and create cohesiveness, and tension may actually promote productivity. The negative aspects of conflict management are that sometimes conflicts suggest a small mind-set of a particular unit rather than promote the good of the whole and sometimes conflict can be carried to the extreme. To resolve a conflict, the manager or leader may function as a mediator, a participant, or a judge. In the participant role, one has to get to the subject of conflict quickly. Try to depersonalize the conflict. Get away from you and I and rather say we. Try to keep feelings low key. Discuss the issue and ways to resolve the conflict. The mediator works as a liaison to get the 2 sides to resolve the conflict. Make suggestions that help both sides. Point out the facts. And remember that, as a mediator, one is an observer and can visualize things through a different pair of lenses. As a judge, the manager or leader will listen to both sides, let both sides have their say and voice their concerns, weigh all facts related to the conflict, and then make a decision.

Some Other Thoughts on Communication

Assertive communication comes from the "I." Rather than the person placing blame on the other party, the individual approaches the subject from his or her own perspective. Aggressive communication is blaming another and pointing the finger at one rather than starting from the "I" perspective. Informal communication is when individuals get together perhaps to discuss things that are related to the work environment. There is no set agenda. One example would be a group of nurse executives from the geographic area getting together quarterly at a dinner just to discuss anything related to life or work but with no set agenda. Persuasive communication occurs all the time when being a manager or leader. If one is in such a position, one has to persuade people to either work an undesirable shift or to work overtime. One also has to consider technology and communication. Has technology really improved the communication process? When we communicate electronically, one major aspect is missing, and that is visualization. We oftentimes cannot see the person as in the communication that is primarily verbal. We cannot pick up on the nonverbal cues of the other party. Another important item to consider is multiculturalism. We have to be sensitive to all cultures in our nation. One patient that I was caring for in the home was 94 years old and was bedbound. She had been a teacher in an elementary school for several years. She looked at my grandson and questioned what nationality he was. He is a combination of about 7 or 8 nationalities. When I explained this to her, she said, "our country is like minestrone soup." I will never forget her words, as they made me realize how many cultures exist in our country and how many Americans have many cultures within their own genes. It is something to consider when we communicate.

To summarize, communication is at the heart of management and leadership. Communication can make or break an institution. Communication is much more than a sender-receiver of information. Thought transmission really is the crux of communication.

CASE EXEMPLAR ON COMMUNICATION

CASE STUDY
Refusal of an Emergency Department Technician to Follow the Direction of a Unit Assistant

John is an EDT (emergency department technician) with a reputation for being slow to complete his assigned tasks. He also "disappears" from the unit and has a negative attitude. One evening the RN Team Leader reported to the Nurse Manager that John refused to transport a patient to computed tomography because he was busy stocking IV carts. The Nurse Manager explained to the RN that he had earlier assigned the EDT to the stocking task because he had just been "sitting around reading." The RN then repeated the patient transporting assignment to the EDT who again refused and sought out the Nurse Manager. In the meantime, the RN Team Leader assigned the transport to another EDT.

John approaches the Nurse Manager with anger in his face and voice. His voice is shaky as he explains, "I do not work for that Team Leader. She has no right to take me from an assignment that you made. If she wants something done she can write it down on a piece of paper and put it in the lab box and I will get to it."

After telling John to lower his voice, I made 2 points: first, patients' needs come first, and second, the RN Team Leader has not only the right but also the responsibility to assign work to the EDTs available on the unit whether they are on her team or not. A peripheral issue is the fact that EDTs are not checking the box in a timely manner, causing patients to needlessly wait. If a patient needs to go to computed tomography, be transferred to a bed upstairs, or have an electrocardiography or other diagnostic procedure, those needs have priority. Furthermore, electrocardiography has to be done no later than 5 minutes after triage.

John continues to argue with the Nurse Manager, especially on the point that not all Team Leaders can tell him and, for that matter, the other EDTs what to do. "All EDTs should report directly to you, the Nurse Manager, and only take orders from you. Besides, I don't like the way the Team Leader orders me around. It's embarrassing!"

He was still frustrated with the situation and wanted all of his assignments written down. The Nurse Manager repeated that the Team Leader's assignment was appropriate and that in the future he needed to honor the fact that patient needs come first. The EDT reluctantly returned to his assignments. Later in the evening, the Nurse Manager asked the Team Leader about her interaction with John. She confessed that she had been sharp with him but that John had been "slacking off" all night and she lost her patience. The Nurse Manager also learned that the other EDTs viewed John as "not pulling his weight." As one EDT put it, "John likes to challenge authority; that is how he gets out of work." The Nurse Manager wrote an extensive corrective action plan for John using the job description of the EDT as the framework. The plan emphasized reporting lines and responsibilities and the fact that patients' needs always come first in the emergency department. John continued to argue during the counseling session but eventually seemed to come to terms with the points made by the Nurse Manager. After 2 weeks, there is an improvement in John's behavior and attitude although he still has a tendency to argue with assignments. The Nurse Manager also met with the RN Team Leaders to discuss the best communication strategies to use when assigning John to tasks and monitoring results.

Questions to Consider

1. What issues are involved in this case?
2. What part does communication play in avoiding or promoting situations of insubordination?
3. Did the Charge Nurse do the correct thing by involving and referring the case to the Assistant Director?
4. How would have you handled this case if you were the Team Leader or the Nurse Manager?

The following algorithm can be used as a management tool for problem-solving this case.

Decision Tree

The following model can be used to decide on an immediate course of action, to plot a course of corrective action, and to recognize leadership principles involved in the case.

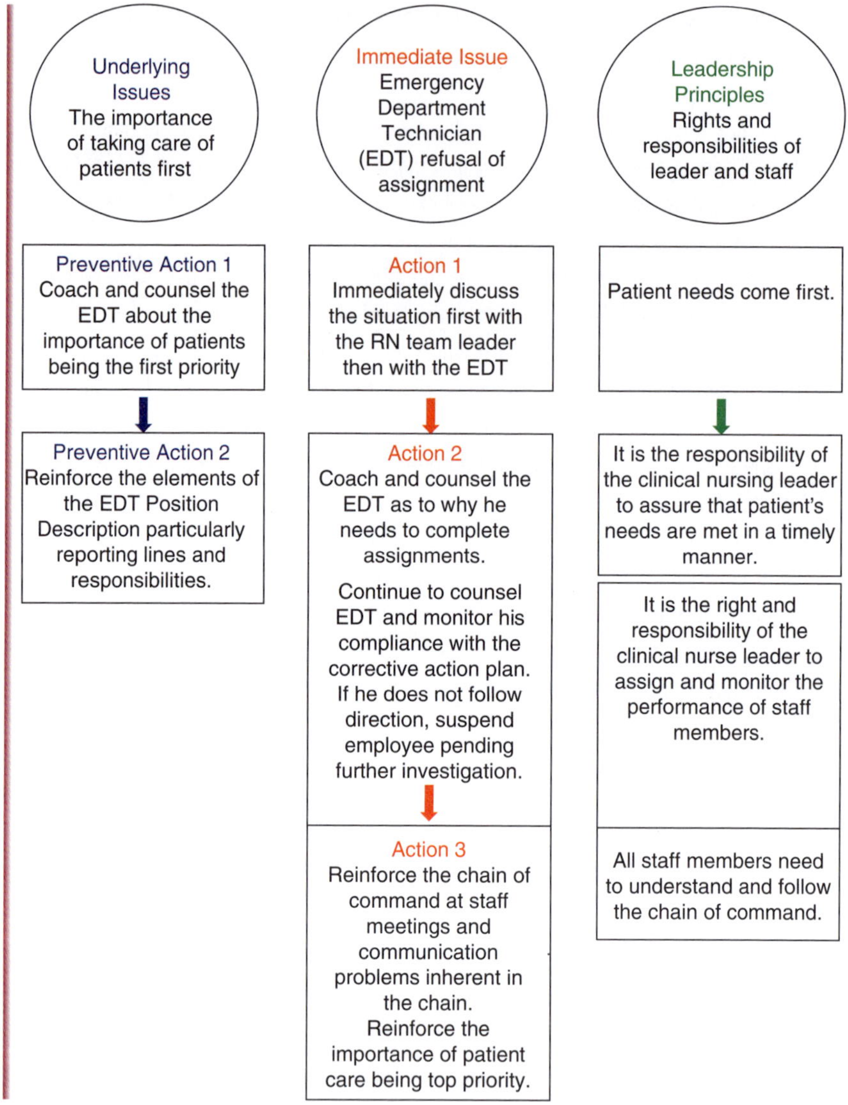

References

Burns, J. (1978). *Leadership*. New York: Harper Row Publishing.

Doody, O., & Doody, C. (2012). Transformational leadership in nursing practice. *British Journal of Nursing, 21*(20), 1212–1218.

Drucker, P. F. (2004). *Critical evaluations in business & management*. New York, New York: Routledge.

Fayol, H. (1949). *General & industrial management*. Translated by C. Storrs. London, England: Sir Isaac Pitman & Sons.

Gosling, J. & Mintzberg, M.(2003). *The five mind of a manager*. Cambridge, Mass: Harvard Business Review.

Hock, D. (2005). *One from many*. San Francisco, CA: Barrett-Koehler Publishers.
Mintzberg, H. (1975). The manager's job: Folklore & fact. Cambridge, Mass: Harvard Business School Press.
Patient Protection & Affordable Care Act. (2010). Retrieved from https://www.thebalance.com/2010-patient-protection-affordable-care-act-3306063.
Salovey, P. & Mayer, J. D. (1990). Emotional intelligence. *Imagination, Cognition & Personality*, 9(3).
Umiker, W. O. (1988). *Management skills for the new health care supervisor*. Aspen Publications.

Resources

American Nurses Association. (2009). *Nursing administration: Scope and standards of practice*. Silver Spring, MD: American Nurses Association.
American Nurses Association. (2015). *Code of ethics with interpretative statements*. Silver Spring, MD: American Nurses Association.
Bonczek, M., & Woodard, E. (August 2006). Who'll replace you when you're gone? *Nursing Management, 37*(8), 30–34. Retrieved June 7, 2008, from Academic Search Premier database.
Chaos Theory for beginners. (n.d.). Retrieved from http://www.abarim-publications.com/ChaosTheoryIntroduction.html#.WUfWNevyt1s.
Definitions of Systems Theory. (n.d.). Retrieved from http://www.cs.unb.ca/profs/fritz/cs3503/system35.htm.
Drucker, P. (2011). *The effective executive*. New York, New York: Routledge Taylor & Francis Group.
Guido, G. W. (2013). *Legal & ethical issues in nursing* (6th ed.). New York City, NY: Pearson Education.
Huber, D. (2010). *Leadership and nursing care management* (4th ed.). Philadelphia: Saunders/Elsevier.
Jones, C. (March 2008). Chief nursing officer retention and turnover: A crisis brewing? Results of a National Survey. *Journal of Healthcare Management, 53*(2), 89–106.
Marshall, E. S., & Broome, M. (2017). *Transformational leadership in nursing*. New York: Springer Publishing.
Mason, D. J., Leavitt, J. K., & Chaffe, M. W. (2007). *Policy & politics in nursing and health care* (5th ed.). St. Louis, MO: W.B. Saunders/Elsevier.
Mason, D. J., Gardner, D. B., Outlaw, F. H., & O'Grady, E. T. (Eds). (2016). *Policy & politics in nursing & health care* (7th ed.). St. Louis, MO: Elsevier.
Mason, W. (n.d.). *Complexity theory*. Retrieved from http://www.referenceforbusiness.com/management/Bun-Comp/Complexity-Theory.html#ixzz4kSTjhNxR.
Melnyk, B., & Fineout-Overholt, E. (2014). *Evidence based practice in nursing and health care* (3rd ed.). Philadelphia, PA: Lippincott.
Page, A. (Ed.). (2004). *Keeping patients safe: Transforming the work environment of nurses*. Washington, DC: Committee on the work environment for nurses and patient safety, Institute of Medicine, National Academies Press.
Polit, D. F., & Beck, C. T. (2017). *Nursing research: Generating and assessing evidence for nursing practice*. Philadelphia, PA: Lippincott.
Rickles, D., Hawe, P., & Shiell, A. (2009). A guide to chaos and complexity. *Journal of Epidemiology and Community Health, 61*(11), 933–937. doi:10.1136/jech.2006.054254.
Roussel, L. (Ed.). (2013). *Management and leadership for nurse administrators*. Burlington, MA: Jones & Bartlett Learning.
Rundio, A. (2012). *Budgeting & finance for nurse managers*. Indianapolis, IN: Sigma Theta Tau Publications.

Rundio, A., & Wilson, V. (Eds.). (2015). *The doctor of nursing practice—the nurse executive role.* Philadelphia, PA: Wolters Kluwer Lippincott.

Rundio, A. (2016a). *Budgeting & finance for nurse managers* (2nd ed.). Indianapolis, IN: Sigma Theta Tau Publications.

Rundio, A. (2016b). *The nurse manager's guide to budgeting & finance* (2nd ed.). Indianapolis, IN: Sigma Theta Tau Publications.

Rundio, A., Wilson V., & Meloy F. (2016). *The nurse executive review and resource manual* (3rd ed.). Silver Spring, MD: ANA Publications.

Showalter, J. S., Southwick, A. F, (1999). *Southwick's the law of health care administration* (3rd ed.). Chicago, IL: Health Administration Press/American College of Health Care Executives.

Witzel, M., & Warner, M. (2013). *The oxford handbook of management theorists.* (Gosling & Mintzberg, pg. 473). United Kingdom: Oxford University Press.

CHAPTER

2

Quality Improvement, Patient Safety, and Risk Management

Frances H. Cornelius

This chapter will review:

QUALITY IMPROVEMENT

STRATEGIES AND APPROACHES FOR QUALITY IMPROVEMENT

TOOLS TO ASSIST WITH QUALITY IMPROVEMENT

THEORIES AND FRAMEWORKS FOR QI AND MANAGING CHANGE

EVALUATION OF CARE DELIVERY OUTCOMES

INTRODUCTION AND OVERVIEW

The American Organization of Nurse Executives (AONE) competencies for nurse executives include skills in quality monitoring and improvement, which requires an in-depth knowledge of systems theories and strategies for continuous quality improvement (QI). The contemporary nurse executive must have a working knowledge of quality improvement and monitoring, strategies to ensure patient safety, and measures to effectively manage and minimize organizational risk. In addition to this knowledge, the effective nurse executive must also possess critical skills—both technical and soft skills—to support these endeavors. These include the ability to (1) create a culture of continuous quality improvement (CQI), (2) translate data into information (including the use of internal and external benchmarks) and disseminate them at various levels within the organization, (3) select the appropriate continuous improvement technique for a given situation, and (4) evaluate outcomes of care delivery (e.g., nursing-sensitive indicators, ORYX indicators, National Patient Safety Goals, Leapfrog, Hospital Consumer Assessment of Healthcare Providers and Systems [HCAHPS]) (AONE, 2015).

QUALITY MONITORING AND IMPROVEMENT

There is no doubt that quality monitoring is essential to improve processes that are inefficient, inconsistent, and fraught with flaws that increase the risk of medical errors. First and foremost, a CQI culture must be fully embraced in a manner in which it is second nature for all team members to reflect on processes and continuously ask questions such as "Is this working?" and "What can we do to improve?" CQI "consists of systematic and continuous actions that lead to measurable improvement in health care services and the health status of targeted patient groups" (U.S. Department of Health and Human Services Health Resources and Services Administration [HRSA], 2011a, 2011b, p. 1). A CQI initiative includes 3 major components, structure, process, and outcomes, which feed back into the structure and process in a continuous loop, driving improvement.

Key Points

- Systematic activities that are "organized and implemented to monitor, assess, and improve its quality of health care" (HRSA, 2011a, p. 5)
- Cyclical activities to permit ongoing pursuit of higher levels of performance to optimize patient care and outcomes (HRSA, 2011a)

To initiate a CQI program, a detailed quality initiative plan must be developed, which has the following properties:

- Provides a detailed work plan for the entire organization's QI activities.
- Provides information regarding "how your organization will manage, deploy, and review quality throughout the organization" (HRSA, 2011b, p. 1).
- Is usually developed by executive and clinical leadership.
- Specifically outlines the specific clinical focus areas for the current and subsequent calendar years.
- Is regularly reviewed and updated.
- Is an iterative process. Data and outcomes from previous years inform development of current and subsequent year's QI plan to reflect "organizational priorities and organizational program requirements" (p. 1).

Wagner et al. (2012) state the following steps to support any CQI initiative:

- Select and use a model or strategy for the continuous quality initiative.
- Identify and regularly monitor outcome metrics.
- Educate staff members regarding the metrics and desired success outcomes.
- Include all stakeholders in the quality initiative activities (patients, families, providers, and health care team).

Key Elements of a Quality Improvement Plan

- Description of organizational mission, program goals, and objectives
- Definition of key quality terms and concepts
- Description of how QI projects are selected, managed, and monitored
- Description of training and support for staff involved in the QI process
- Description of quality methodology (such as Plan-Do-Study-Act [PDSA], Exit Disclaimer, Six Sigma Exit Disclaimer) and quality tools and techniques to be used throughout the organization
- Description of the communication plan of planned QI activities and processes and how updates will be communicated to the management and staff on a regular basis
- Description of measurement and analysis and how it will help define future QI activities
- Description of evaluation and quality assurance activities that will be used to determine the effectiveness of the QI plan's implementation (HRSA, 2011b, p. 2)

Strategies for Continuous Quality Improvement

There are many strategies that can be used to improve quality and safety within a health care organization. In this section, several approaches for ensuring CQI in health care are described, including PDSA, The Model for Improvement, Lean, Six Sigma, Root Cause Analysis (RCA), 5 Whys, and 5 Hows.

Plan-Do-Study-Act

The PDSA cycle is a practical and systematic approach for documenting a test of a change within a system. The steps in the cycle include (1) Plan: the development of a plan to test a change; (2) Do: the actual testing of the change; (3) Study: observing, analyzing, and learning from the test; and (4) Act: determining if any modifications are needed for the next cycle of the PDSA.

The cycle is first applied as a pilot and repeated until it is determined that no further modifications are needed, and then the scale of the cycle is increased until it is considered appropriate to implement a wide-scale change. Data from each cycle are used to inform and drive subsequent testing cycles, leading to improved results (see Figure 2.1).

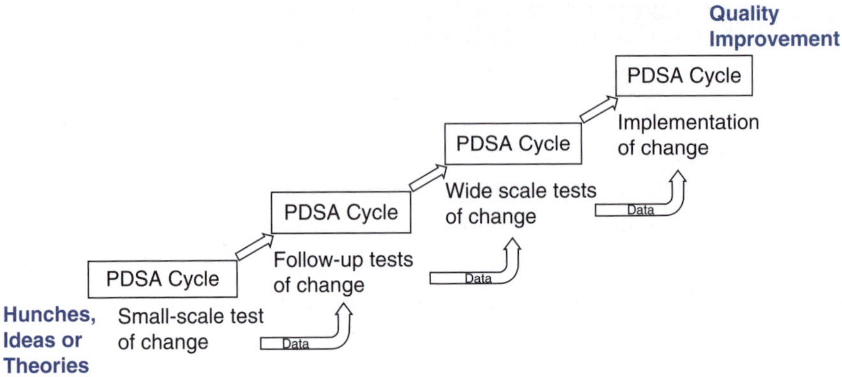

FIGURE 2.1 The Plan-Do-Study-Act (PDSA) cycle for quality improvement. (Adapted from Associates in Process Improvement. Retrieved from http://www.apiweb.org/index.php.)

Key Points

- Walter A. Shewhart developed the Plan-Do-Check-Act cycle.
- W. Edwards Deming modified Shewhart's cycle to PDSA, replacing "Check" with "Study."
- The PDSA cycle is also referred to as the "Deming cycle."
- Although the PDSA cycle is iterative, it is important to do the steps in order.
- Include both internal and external stakeholders.
- Communicate accomplishments to internal and external customers.
- Take steps to preserve your gains and sustain your accomplishments.
- Make long-term plans for additional improvements.

The Model for Improvement

The Model for Improvement, developed by Associates in Process Improvement, is an expansion of the PDSA model and provides a very effective tool for accelerating improvement (Associates in Process Improvement [API], 2017). In 1994, Langley et al. suggested that the use of PDSA cycles would be more effective if 3 questions are considered before using each PDSA cycle (Langley, Nolan, Nolan, Norman, & Provost, 2009). As a result, the Model for Improvement has 2 main components: (1) 3 fundamental questions and (2) the PDSA cycle (Institute for Healthcare Improvement [IHI], 2017b).

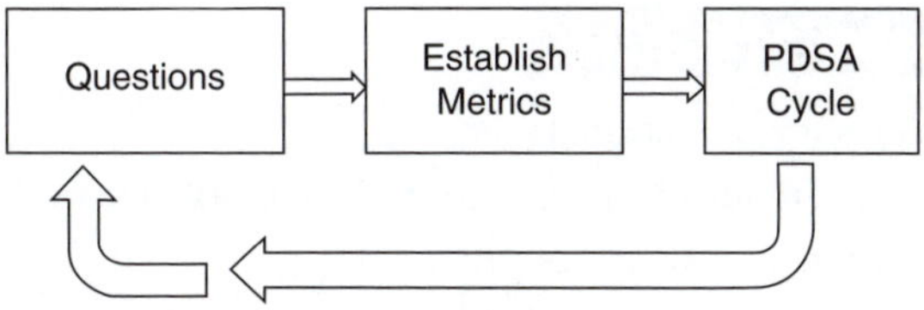

FIGURE 2.2 Institute for Healthcare Improvement (IHI) model for improvement.

Key Points (IHI, 2017a, 2017b, 2017c, 2017d)

- The questions to ask:
  - What are we trying to accomplish?
  - How will we know that a change is an improvement?
  - What change can we make that will result in an improvement?
- The questions can be answered in any order.
- Metrics: Goals/aims should be measurable, be time specific, and clearly convey who or what is being measured.
- Measures are quantitative.
- The PDSA cycle should be first "tested" on a small scale to permit assessing change effectiveness and providing opportunity to refine the change before implementing on a large scale (dissemination) (Figure 2.2).

Lean

Lean is a CQI approach that emphasizes the focus on customer value and minimizing waste of resources. The Lean approach considers 3 factors that are central to all organizations: (1) Purpose, (2) Process, and (3) People. The key goal of Lean is to gain operational efficiency while maintaining and improving customer value, specifically "reducing non–value-added activities, mistake-proofing tasks, and relentlessly focusing on reducing waste to improve health care delivery. Lean helps operationalize the change to create work flows, handoffs, and processes that work over the long term" (NLC, 2013, p. 10).

The Lean approach focuses on changes that improve operations, specifically changes that reduce waste. Levinson and Rerick (2002) identify 7 kinds of waste: (1) overproduction, (2) waiting time (time in queue), (3) transportation, (4) non–value-adding processes, (5) inventory, (6) motion, and (7) costs of quality, scrap, rework, and inspection.

Key Points (NLC, 2013, p. 11)

- Lean principles for operational efficiency:
  - Identify value: in terms of value from the clients' viewpoint; in terms that are specific to the service provided.
  - Specify value: map the steps that bring the service or product to the client. Include both value-added steps and non–value-added steps.
  - Workflow process: focus on CQI of processes, services, and information flow from start to finish through the entire cycle.
  - Push/pull activities: integrate clients' requirements/specifications into upstream processes.
  - Process delivery: promote CQI efforts through elimination of wasteful, non–value-added activities.
- Lean CQI focuses on elimination of waste, overburden, and inconsistency.
- Internal and external perspectives provide insight in determining value.
- Value stream is the sequence of activities that contribute to value.
- Activities that do not contribute to value (non–value added) are waste and should be eliminated or streamlined.
- Focus should be on improving the flow of value-added activities and information to ensure efficient processes.
- Test flow of processes to ensure that processes have improved and perfect the process.

Six Sigma

Six Sigma is also a model that has its origins in business with the goal of improving efficiency, eliminating causes of defects/errors, and maximizing consistency of manufacturing and business processes. Specifically, "Six Sigma is a disciplined, data-driven approach and methodology for eliminating defects (driving toward six standard deviations between the mean and the nearest specification limit) in any process – from manufacturing to transactional and from product to service" (iSixSigma, 2017b, ¶ 1). This approach uses 2 submethodologies. The first, DMAIC, includes 5 steps: (1) define, (2) measure, (3) analyze, (4) improve, and (5) control while also applying statistical modeling and quality management methods to system improvement endeavors. The approach relies heavily on data, process, and outcome measures. Six Sigma methodologies are often used in tandem with Lean and is a particularly effective combination when the goal is to reduce waste and errors.

Key Points (iSixSigma, 2017a, 2017b)

- Initially when Six Sigma was developed, it functioned as a scale for levels of quality; for example, Six Sigma refers to 6 defects per 1 million opportunities.
- It is purely a data-driven process for QI.
- Focus is on process improvement and variation reduction through the application of Six Sigma improvement projects.
- There are 3 levels of Six Sigma certification: (1) green belt, (2) black belt, and (3) master black belt.
- Both Green and Black Belts can execute Six Sigma improvement projects.
- Improvement projects are overseen by black belts.
- Improvement projects use 1 of the 2 submethodologies: DMAIC and DMADV.
- Both submethodologies appear to be linear approaches, but are, in fact, very fluid.
- Although the acronyms seem similar, the methods are distinctly different.
  - DMAIC
    - Components: define, measure, analyze, improve, control (Figure 2.3).
    - Process improvement approach for existing processes that need improvement.
    - The DMAIC method is used "when a product or process is in existence at your company but is not meeting customer specification or is not performing adequately" (iSixSigma, 2017a, ¶ 4).
  - DMADV
    - Components: define, measure, analyze, design, verify (Figure 2.4).
    - Systematic approach to develop new processes or products at quality levels.
    - The DMADV method is used when:
      - "A product or process is not in existence at your company and one needs to be developed.
      - The existing product or process exists and has been optimized (using either DMAIC or not) and still does not meet the level of customer specification or Six Sigma level" (iSixSigma, 2017a, ¶ 6).

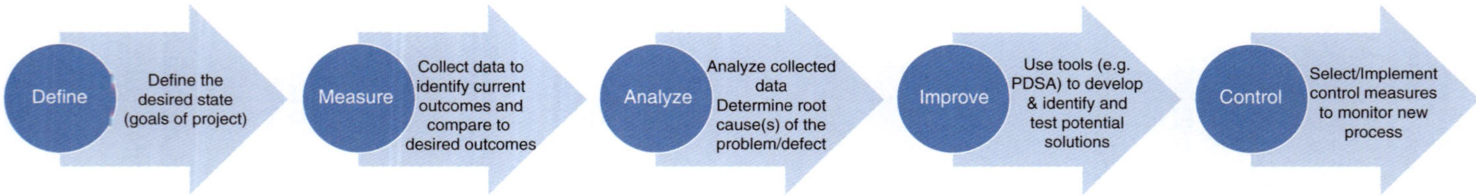

FIGURE 2.3 Six Sigma DMAIC (define, measure, analyze, improve, and control) quality improvement approach.

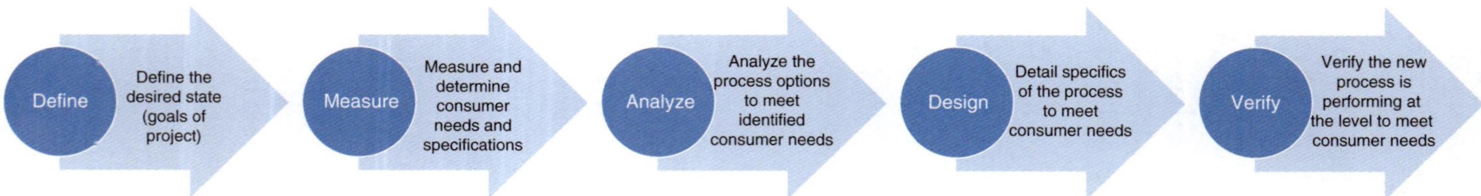

FIGURE 2.4 Six Sigma DMADV (define, measure, analyze, design, verify) quality improvement approach.

Root Cause Analysis

RCA is a systematic approach to examine a negative event to identify contributing factors that directly caused the event. RCA is also referred to as the "5 Whys." Contributing factors are process or system issues that can lead to the negative event. Root causes are defined as "underlying faulty process or system issues that lead to the harmful event" (Centers for Medicare and Medicaid Services [CMS], n.d., p. 6). Frequently, there is more than one root cause for an event. Sakichi Toyada is credited with the development of this approach (Bialek, Duffy, & Moran, 2009; Quality-One International, 2015).

Key Points

- This process is a reactive approach rather than a proactive approach, analyzing factors contributing to something that has happened.
- It can be proactive in that it can be used to prevent future failures or negative outcomes, but it is not primarily a proactive approach.
- It takes a deeper look at underlying factors rather than the obvious cause.
- RCA is also referred to as the "5 Whys."

It is not always necessary to ask "Why" 5 times. The intent is to get you to dig deep enough to uncover the true root cause of the negative event; however, it is essential that the RCA analysis technique be used appropriately. It is recommended that the following steps be followed when doing an RCA:

1. Factually describe and document the whole event.
2. Gather the evidence to support your description of the event.
3. Classify your evidence along a proper timeline in which the events occurred ending with the final failure.
4. Identify the causes by asking "why" along each step. Remember the 5 Whys method.
5. Separate root causes along each step that affected the event in any way from the casual causes without direct impact on the final failure.
6. Identify all possible preventive measures and place them in order with the simplest and most cost-effective measure at the top.
7. Classify these measures further by identifying the ones that have a group consensus and are likely to have the highest possible rate of preventing the problem in the future without creating other disturbances.

8. Seek any other methods necessary to reach the root cause depending on the complexity of your problem and field.
9. Apply these corrective measures to ensure future prevention and safety (Fatima, 2015, ¶ 22).

The 5 Hows

After completing the *5 Whys*, the *5 Hows* method is used to identify a "permanent solution to the "root cause (s)" of the problem" (Quality-One International, 2015, ¶ 3).

Used in combination, the 5 Whys and 5 Hows "constitute a questioning process designed to drill down into the details of a problem or a solution and peel away the layers of symptoms" (Bialek et al., 2009, p. 168).

Key Considerations for Ensuring Success

Groene, Kringos, and Sunol (2014) identify 7 strategies for success with an organizational QI initiative:

1. Monitor and adapt to the external environment to ensure alignment.
2. Prioritize quality and communicate that throughout the organization.
3. Establish organizational systems and infrastructure to support and sustain QI.
4. Place right people with expertise with responsibilities at department level.
5. Use evidence quality and safety evidence to establish processes and pathways.
6. "Implement pathway-oriented information systems.
7. Conduct regular assessment and provide feedback" (p. 5).

Tools for Quality Improvement Projects

In this section, these tools are reviewed and key characteristics described. There are several tools that can support QI projects. The IHI provides a Quality Improvement Essentials Toolkit that is available on their Web site and includes an overview of the top tools with templates to use in a QI project (IHI, 2017a, 2017b, 2017c, 2017d). In addition, Health Resources and Services Administration also has a wide variety of resources in its Quality Toolbox. Links to these resources are listed at the end of the chapter.

Cause and Effect Diagram

Also known as the Ishikawa diagram, a cause and effect diagram is an organizational tool that graphically presents cause and effect relationships to help teams explore the factors contributing to a certain effect or outcome (IHI, 2017a).

Key Characteristics (American Society for Quality, 2017a; IHI, 2017a)

- Using the cause and effect diagram helps identify the cause of the problem.
- Key question to ask is, "Why does this happen?" and to continue to ask is "Why?" until deeper causes are identified.
- Graphic display helps identify areas for improvement.
- This is also known as a fishbone diagram, because of its resemblance to the bones of a fish.
- Factors contributing to an effect or outcome are grouped in the categories of Materials, Methods, Equipment, Environment, and People.

Driver Diagram

A driver diagram is an effective tool that can provide a visual display of drivers (contributing factors) that support the attainment of a project goal. "A driver diagram shows the relationship between the overall aim of the project, the primary drivers (sometimes called "key drivers") that contribute directly to achieving the aim, the secondary drivers that are components of the primary drivers, and specific change ideas to test for each secondary driver" (IHI, 2017a, p.7).

Key Characteristics (National Health Service Institute for Innovation and Improvement, 2011)

- A clearly defined goal/aim is essential; ideally it should be measurable.
- Primary drivers are the most important influencers on the goal/aim.
- Secondary and tertiary drivers are influencers/subcomponents of the primary drivers.
- All drivers should be measurable.
- This is a team activity; working as a team to identify drivers ensures that all drivers within a complex system are identified.

Failure Modes and Effects Analysis

Failure Modes and Effects Analysis (FMEA) is a proactive method to identify all the possible failures that could occur in the design, system process, pathway, or final product or outcome and to determine the effects of these failures. The FMEA steps are as follows:

- "Failure modes (What could go wrong?)
- Failure causes (Why would the failure happen?)
- Failure effects (What would be the consequences of each failure?)" (IHI, 2017c, ¶ 2)

The American Society for Quality (ASQ) identifies 6 situations in which an FMEA approach should be used:

- "When a process, product, or service is being designed or redesigned, after quality function deployment
- When an existing process, product, or service is being applied in a new way
- Before developing control plans for a new or modified process
- When improvement goals are planned for an existing process, product, or service
- When analyzing failures of an existing process, product, or service
- Periodically throughout the life of the process, product, or service" (2017c, ¶ 8)

Key Characteristics

- FMEA is considered one of the most efficient ways to identify potential failures early in the development cycle.
- Key value added is that FMEA provides the ability to anticipate problems early.
- It permits "design out" failures and "design in" reliable, safe processes/features.

Flowchart

A flowchart provides a visual representation of a workflow or process in sequential order. A flowchart includes a "sequence of actions, materials or services entering or leaving the process (inputs and outputs), decisions that must be made, people who become involved, time involved at each step and/or process measurements" (ASQ, 2017d, ¶ 4). A flowchart should be used

- To develop understanding of how a process is done
- To study a process for improvement
- To communicate to others how a process is done

- When better communication is needed between people involved with the same process
- To document a process
- When planning a project (ASQ, 2017d, ¶ 6)

Key Characteristics

- A flowchart must involve all key people involved in the process.
- Development of a flowchart often requires team effort, as few people would know every aspect of a process.
- People involved in the process should create the flowchart.
- "Variations:
  - macro flowchart,
  - top-down flowchart,
  - detailed flowchart (also called process map, micro map, service map, or symbolic flowchart),
  - deployment flowchart (also called down-across or cross-functional flowchart),
  - several-leveled flowchart" (ASQ, 2017d, ¶ 2).

Histogram

A histogram is a type of bar graph that visually presents continuous data (such as time, weight, size, temperature) chunked in intervals to make it easier to see patterns that are occurring. "A histogram enables a team to recognize and analyze patterns in data that are not apparent simply by looking at a table of data, or by finding the average or median" (IHI, 2017d, ¶ 2). For example, consider Table 2.1.

The data table may reveal to you that, of 32 stress tests that were performed at your institution, the average turnaround time for the final report to get into the medical record was 8.3 days. This is interesting and something to examine more closely. Consider the histogram in Figure 2.5.

The histogram can display this information in a manner that more clearly highlights areas of concern—specifically that although 40% of the reports are finalized within 1 to 2 days, **31% of the reports take 13 to 20 days to get back to the patient's record**—something that needs to be addressed from a quality perspective (Figure 2.6). The histogram presents this information effectively.

Pareto Chart

The Pareto chart is a bar chart in which "factors that contribute to an overall effect are arranged in order from the largest to the smallest contribution to

TABLE 2.1 Stress Test Results Turnaround Time in Days

Test Turnaround Time in Days				Total Turnaround Time/Tests
9	16	1	4	30/4
15	8	13	1	37/4
13	16	14	17	60/4
7	10	20	2	39/4
2	2	18	3	25/4
1	10	2	7	21/4
1	2	15	2	20/4
Total days/number of tests				232/28
Average Turnaround Time in Days				8.3 days

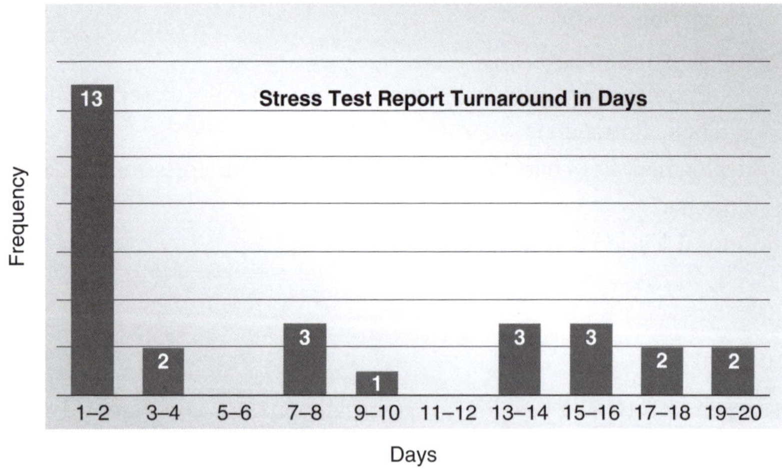

FIGURE 2.5 Stress test report histogram.

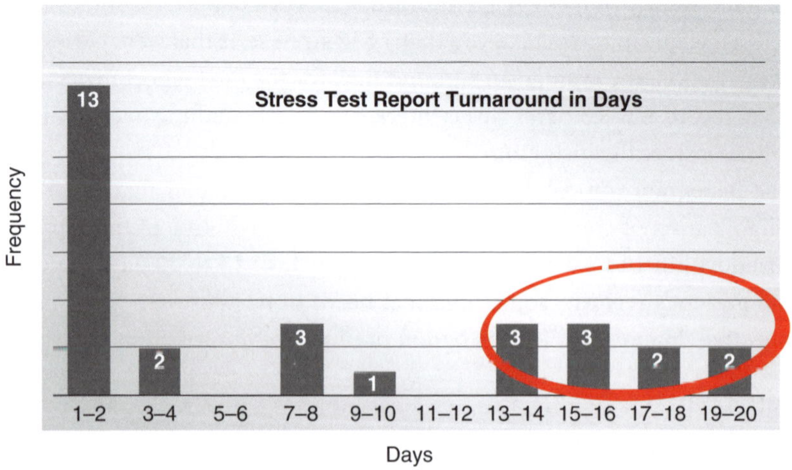

FIGURE 2.6 Stress report turnaround concern area.

the effect. This ordering helps identify the "vital few" (the factors that have the largest contribution to the effect and therefore warrant the most attention), as distinguished from the "useful many" (factors that, while useful to know about, have a relatively smaller contribution to the effect)" (IHI, 2017a, p.27).

Key Characteristics (American Society for Quality, 2017e; IHI, 2017a)

- The Pareto chart is also known as the 80/20 rule that maintains that among any group of factors/causes that contribute to an effect/problem, approximately 80% of the effect/problem comes from 20% of the factors/causes (IHI, 2017a).
- Data are collected first using a simple data table, listing all the factors and the number of occurrences.
- Data are then organized and displayed as a bar graph representing factors that contribute to an effect/problem.
- Data are arranged as the largest bar (greatest number of occurrences) to the smallest (least/insignificant occurrences) to visually represent the factors that contribute the most to the effect/problem.
- This allows QI teams to focus on the factors/causes that have the greatest impact on the problem they are seeking to improve.

Run Chart and Control Chart

A run chart is a graph that provides a visual representation of data collected over time to monitor an area of concern, such as infection rates (Figure 2.7). This is a very effective and easy-to-use tool to conduct ongoing monitoring to see if desired QIs are occurring (IHI, 2017a).

A control chart is a run chart that includes upper control and lower control limits so that it is easier to distinguish normal variances from special-cause variances that are occurring. For example, in Figure 2.8, April and August would be identified as special-cause variances.

Scatter Diagram

A scatter diagram or scatter plot is used when examining 2 variables that may have a cause and effect relationship. Scatter diagrams are often used after a cause and effect diagram has been completed. QI teams may wish to explore more deeply whether a correlation exists between 2 variables (American Society for Quality, 2017b; IHI, 2017a).

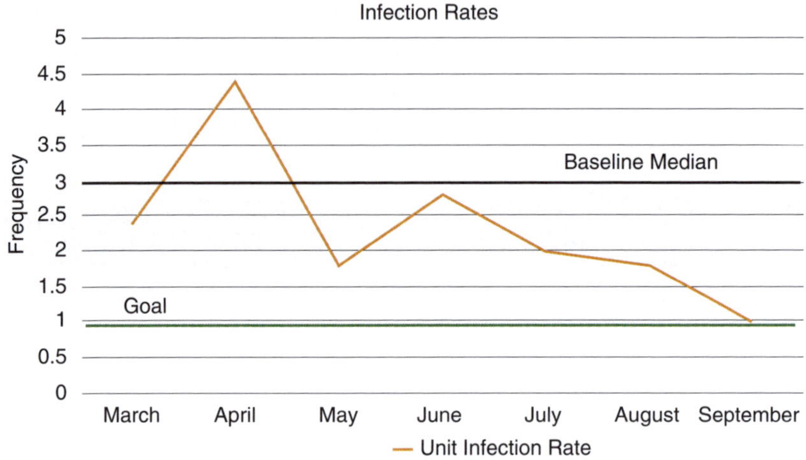

FIGURE 2.7 Run chart depicting infection rate improvement over time.

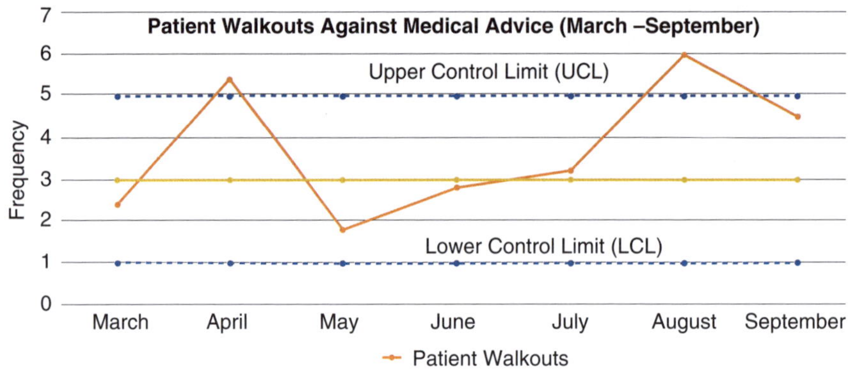

FIGURE 2.8 Control chart depicting normal variance versus special-cause variance.

Key Characteristics

- It is a typical X-Y graph that displays paired numerical data.
- If correlation exists, data points on the graph will present as a line or curve.
- Use a "Scatter diagram:
  - When you have paired numerical data.
  - When your dependent variable may have multiple values for each value of your independent variable.
  - When trying to determine whether the two variables are related" (American Society for Quality, 2017b, ¶ 2).

Deming's System of Profound Knowledge

It would be remiss not to include W. Edwards Deming's contribution to quality and safety initiatives in this chapter. Deming is known for his transformative management philosophy, which has had a profound impact on manufacturing and service organizations on a global scale and changed how we think about quality, management, and leadership. Deming's theory of management and his *System of Profound Knowledge (SoPK)* represent a holistic approach to leadership and management. The philosophy brings together an understanding of variation, theory of knowledge, psychology and appreciation for a system" (The W. Edwards Deming Institute, 2017a, ¶ 2).

Key Points

- The SoPK approach provides a mechanism for people and organizations to continually improve.
- A leader must have a deep understanding of the system that he or she is managing (Martin, n.d.).
- It explores system causes of variances rather than human factors.

Deming also put forth 14 Points of Management, which are listed in Table 2.2. Some text is bolded intentionally to emphasize the elements that relate directly to QI and safety.

Systems Theories

Various system theories can assist the nurse leader in examining and understanding his or her organization. They are described and discussed within the context of the human body. Using systems theory as a framework can be helpful when striving to implement QI endeavors and when facilitating sustainable changes in organizations. In this section, general systems theory, chaos theory, and complex adaptive systems are reviewed.

General Systems Theory

General systems theory was developed by a biologist named Ludwig von Bertalanffy. It refers to "a general science of 'wholeness'" and includes as a foundational premise that "systems" of various orders present as "phenomena not resolvable into local events, dynamic interactions manifest in the difference of behavior of parts when isolated or in a higher configuration…" and "are not

TABLE 2.2. Deming's 14 Points of Management

1. **Create constancy of purpose toward improvement of product and service, with the aim to become competitive and to stay in business, and to provide jobs.**
2. Adopt the new philosophy. We are in a new economic age. Western management must awaken to the challenge, must learn their responsibilities, and take on leadership for change.
3. **Cease dependence on inspection to achieve quality. Eliminate the need for inspection on a mass basis by building quality into the product in the first place.**
4. End the practice of awarding business on the basis of price tag. Instead, minimize total cost. Move toward a single supplier for any one item, on a long-term relationship of loyalty and trust.
5. **Improve constantly and forever the system of production and service, to improve quality and productivity, and thus constantly decrease costs.**
6. Institute training on the job.
7. Institute leadership. The aim of supervision should be to help people and machines and gadgets to do a better job. Supervision of management is in need of overhaul, as well as supervision of production workers.
8. Drive out fear so that everyone may work effectively for the company.
9. Break down barriers between departments. People in research, design, sales, and production must work as a team, to foresee problems of production and in use that may be encountered with the product or service.
10. Eliminate slogans, exhortations, and targets for the work force asking for zero defects and new levels of productivity. Such exhortations only create adversarial relationships, as the bulk of the causes of low quality and low productivity belong to the system and thus lie beyond the power of the work force.
    a. Eliminate work standards (quotas) on the factory floor. Substitute leadership.
    b. Eliminate management by objective. Eliminate management by numbers and numerical goals. Substitute leadership.
11. Remove barriers that rob the hourly worker of his right to pride of workmanship. **The responsibility of supervisors must be changed from sheer numbers to quality.**
12. Remove barriers that rob people in management and in engineering of their right to pride of workmanship. This means, inter alia, abolishment of the annual or merit rating and of management by objective.
13. **Institute a vigorous program of education and self-improvement.**
14. **Put everybody in the company to work to accomplish the transformation. The transformation is everybody's job.**

From Deming WE. Out of the Crisis: 14 Points. 1st ed. Cambridge, Mass.: MIT Press; 2000:23-24.

understandable by investigation of their respective parts in isolation" (Von Bertalanffy, 1968, p. 37). In short, you cannot understand a system if you are only examining a part of the system.

Key Points Regarding General Systems Theory

- GST integrates various sciences (e.g., natural sciences, social sciences).
- It applies universal principles to systems in general.
- It consists of 2 types of systems: closed systems and open systems.
  - A closed system is isolated from its environment.
  - An open system interacts with its environment.
- Complex systems may include a combination of open and closed systems (Cordon, 2013).

Complex Adaptive Systems

Complex adaptive systems are characterized by "various levels of hierarchies, networks, and layers of complexities, have the ability to learn to adapt to its changing components and environment" (Cordon, 2013, p.17).

Key Characteristics of a Complex Adaptive System

- Interactions of the system components are complex, nonlinear, and diverse.
- The system has the capacity to "learn" and adapt (react) in response to the feedback or input from the external environment.
- It is responsive to system changes or changes in the environment.
- It can adapt and be proactive through "self-organization, learning, and reasoning," in response to change (Cordon, 2013, p.17).

Chaos Theory

The chaos theory is used to describe the relationship between order and chaos and to explain how organic systems respond to change. "One of the underlying principles in chaos theory is the notion that there is order that emerge out of chaos, and that everything is interrelated. In systems with interconnected networks, slight disturbances in one part of the system may create major changes far from where they originate" (Cordon, 2013, p. 17–18).

Evaluating Outcomes of Care Delivery

A nurse executive must possess skills in evaluating outcomes of care delivery using a variety of outcome measures, including nursing-sensitive indicators, ORYX indicators, National Patient Safety Goals, Leapfrog, and HCAHPS. Earlier in this chapter, QI methods, approaches, and tools were reviewed. These can be used to capture outcome data using desired outcome measures.

Nursing-Sensitive Indicators

Nursing-sensitive indicators fall into 3 distinct categories: structure, process, and outcome. "Nursing-sensitive indicators identify structures of care and care processes, both of which in turn influence care outcomes. Nursing-sensitive indicators are distinct and specific to nursing, and differ from medical indicators of care quality" (Montalvo, 2007, ¶ 4).

- An example of a nursing-sensitive structure indicator is the nurse vacancy rate.
- An example of a nursing-sensitive process indicator is pain assessment and subsequent reassessment.
- An example of a nursing-sensitive outcome indicator is hospital-acquired infection rate.

ORYX Indicators

The Joint Commission's ORYX Performance Measurement Initiative provides guidance and support to Commission accredited organizations, and those seeking accreditation, in QI endeavors. As part of this initiative, The Joint Commission identifies select vendors as ORYX vendors that can support organizations in collecting performance outcome data. An ORYX vendor provides the following:

- Processes for collecting and analyzing measure data from multiple organizations, as well as disseminating the results of analysis to its client base
- An automated database that can be used to facilitate performance improvement in health care organizations
- The ability to generate both internal comparisons of each participating organization's performance over time and external comparisons of performance among participating organizations
- The ability to transmit data for a specified period (The Joint Commission, February 16, 2017, ¶ 1)

Key Characteristics

- The term oryx refers to a "a swiftly moving and graceful gazelle-like animal" to reflect the importance of an organization to be nimble and responsive to its environment.
- ORYX "incorporates the reporting on performance measure data into its accreditation and certification processes" (The Joint Commission, February 16, 2017, ¶ 2).
- It is intended to support Joint Commission "accredited and -certified organizations in their quality improvement efforts" (The Joint Commission, February 16, 2017, ¶ 2).
- ORYX data are available to the public on The Joint Commission Web site at www.qualitycheck.org.
- The performance measure data are publicly available and permit user comparisons of hospital performance on individual measures at the state and national levels (The Joint Commission, February 16, 2017, ¶ 2).

National Patient Safety Goals

The Joint Commission's National Patient Safety Goals program focuses on patient safety in 8 main care delivery areas: (1) ambulatory health care, (2) behavioral health care, (3) critical access hospital, (4) home care, (5) hospital, (6) laboratory safety, (7) nursing care center, and (8) office-based surgery safety. Specific goals for each area are listed in Table 2.3.

Leapfrog Group

The Leapfrog Group is a "nonprofit watchdog organization that serves as a voice for health care purchasers, using their collective influence to foster positive change in U.S. health care. Leapfrog is the nation's premier advocate of hospital transparency—collecting, analyzing, and disseminating hospital data" (Leapfrog, n.d.). The intent is to support the development of an informed health care consumer. The Leapfrog Group collects information about hospitals and physicians as well as other metrics. The following are the specific outcome reports available through the Leapfrog Group:

- Basic hospital information
- Medication safety—computerized physician order entry
- Inpatient surgery
- Maternity care

TABLE 2.3. National Patient Safety Goals for Care Delivery Areas

Safety in ambulatory health care • Identify patients correctly • Use medicines safely • Prevent infection • Prevent mistakes in surgery	Safety in behavioral health care • Identify individuals served correctly • Use medications safely • Prevent infection • Identify individuals served safety risks
Safety in critical access hospital • Identify patients correctly • Prevent infection • Use alarms safely • Improve staff communication • Use medicines safely • Prevent mistakes in surgery	Safety in home care • Identify patients correctly • Prevent infection • Prevent patients from falling • Identify patient safety risks • Use medicines safely
Safety in the hospital • Identify patients correctly • Prevent infection • Improve staff communication • Identify patient safety risks • Prevent mistakes in surgery	Nursing care center safety • Identify residents correctly • Use medicines safely • Prevent infection • Prevent residents from falling • Prevent bed sores
Laboratory safety • Identify patients correctly • Improve staff communication • Prevent infection	Office-based surgery safety • Identify patients correctly • Use medicine safely • Prevent infection • Prevent mistakes in surgery

- ICU physician staffing
- National Quality Forum safe practices
- Managing serious errors
- Medication safety
- Pediatric care

Hospital Consumer Assessment of Healthcare Providers and Systems

"Hospital Consumer Assessment of Healthcare Providers and Systems (HCAHPS) survey is the first national, standardized, publicly reported survey of patients' perspectives of their hospital experience" (Center for Medicare and Medicaid Services [CMS], 2009, p. 1).

Key Characteristics

- The survey permits valid comparisons across hospitals locally, regionally, and nationally.
- It is designed to produce data about patients' perspectives of care that allow objective and meaningful comparisons of hospitals on topics that are important to consumers.
- Survey results create new incentives for hospitals to improve quality of care.
- The survey enhances accountability in health care by increasing transparency of the quality of hospital care provided in return for the public investment.

QUALITY AND SAFETY EDUCATION FOR NURSES

The Quality and Safety Education for Nurses (QSEN) project has the broad goal of meeting the "challenge of preparing future nurses who will have the knowledge, skills and attitudes (KSAs) necessary to continuously improve the quality and safety of the healthcare systems within which they work" (QSEN, 2017).

QSEN competencies were drawn from the Institute of Medicine competencies and developed by the QSEN faculty and a National Advisory Board. There are QSEN competencies for prelicensure programs and for graduate nursing programs. Both prelicensure and graduate competencies have 6 categories presented in Table 2.4.

TABLE 2.4. Quality and Safety Education for Nurses (QSEN) Competency Domains with Definitions

QSEN Competency Domain	Definition
Patient-centered care	Recognize the patient or designee as the source of control and full partner in providing compassionate and coordinated care based on respect for patient's preferences, values, and needs.
Teamwork and collaboration	Function effectively within nursing and interprofessional teams, fostering open communication, mutual respect, and shared decision making to achieve quality patient care.
Evidence-based practice	Integrate best current evidence with clinical expertise and patient/family preferences and values for delivery of optimal health care.

(Continued)

TABLE 2.4. Quality and Safety Education for Nurses (QSEN) Competency Domains with Definitions—cont'd

QSEN Competency Domain	Definition
Quality improvement	Use data to monitor the outcomes of care processes and use improvement methods to design and test changes to continuously improve the quality and safety of health care systems.
Safety	Minimize risk of harm to patients and providers through both system effectiveness and individual performance.
Informatics	Use information and technology to communicate, manage knowledge, mitigate error, and support decision making.

QSEN Institute (2017). *QSEN competencies.* Available from: http://qsen.org/competencies/pre-licensure-ksas/#quality_improvement. Reproduced with permission from Quality and Safety Education for Nurses (QSEN).

QUESTIONS

1. To accelerate improvement when using a PDSA mode for improvement, the nurse manager would ask which of the following questions?
   a. What are the available resources?
   b. What are the changes we want to make?
   c. How will we know that a change is an improvement?
   d. Who should be involved?
2. Which of the following statements regarding the RCA process is not correct?
   a. It is a reactive approach.
   b. It is a proactive approach.
   c. It can identify multiple contributing factors.
   d. It can help identify faulty system issues.
3. A nurse manager is planning to create a driver diagram to depict drivers that can support a QI project and present this to the executive leadership team at an upcoming meeting. His or her presentation will be effective if he or she does all of the following except:
   a. Finishes the diagram himself or herself in time for the meeting
   b. Identifies the primary drivers
   c. Includes secondary and tertiary drivers as influencers/subcomponents of the primary drivers
   d. Lists drivers as measurable terms

4. You want to examine a negative event to identify contributing factors that directly caused the event. The best approach to do this is:
   a. Workflow diagram
   b. The DMADV technique
   c. The 5 Hows
   d. PDSA
5. The Lean approach focuses on changes that improve operations and specifically reduce waste in all except which of the following?
   a. Overproduction
   b. Time in queue
   c. Value-adding processes
   d. Motion
6. The best way to display continuous data collected over time is a:
   a. Scatter chart
   b. Run chart
   c. Histogram
   d. Control chart
7. FMEA is a proactive method to identify possible failures. An FMEA approach should be used in which of the following situations?
   a. When a process, product, or service is being redistributed
   b. When an existing process, product, or service is being used
   c. Before developing control plans for a new or modified process
   d. When improvement goals are being monitored
8. Which of the following theories would view an organization as a system characterized by various levels of hierarchies and networks?
   a. General systems theory
   b. Organizational theory
   c. Complex adaptive systems
   d. Chaos theory
9. Metrics for QI projects must be all of the following except:
   a. Measurable
   b. Qualitative
   c. Time specific
   d. Clear
10. The best way to display data collected over time and distinguish normal variances from special-cause variances is a:
   a. Scatter chart
   b. Run chart
   c. Histogram
   d. Control chart
11. To examine the medication administration process within the hospital, which tool would you use?
   a. Histogram
   b. Flowchart
   c. Driver diagram
   d. Cause and effect diagram

ANSWERS: 1-c, 2-b, 3-a, 4-c, 5-c, 6-c, 7-c, 8-c, 9-b, 10-d, 11-b

References

American Organization of Nurse Executives. (2015). *AONE nurse executive competencies*. Chicago, IL: American Organization of Nurse Executives. Retrieved from http://www.aone.org/resources/nurse-leader-competencies.shtml.

American Society for Quality. (2017a). *Cause analysis tools: Fishbone diagram*. Retrieved from http://www.asq.org/learn-about-quality/cause-analysis-tools/overview/fishbone.html.

American Society for Quality. (2017b). *Scatter diagram*. Retrieved from http://asq.org/learn-about-quality/cause-analysis-tools/overview/scatter.html.

American Society for Quality. (2017c). *Failure modes and effects analysis (FMEA)*. Retrieved from http://asq.org/learn-about-quality/process-analysis-tools/overview/fmea.html.

American Society for Quality. (2017d). *What is a process flowchart?* Retrieved from http://asq.org/learn-about-quality/process-analysis-tools/overview/flowchart.html.

American Society for Quality. (2017e). *Pareto chart*. Retrieved from http://asq.org/learn-about-quality/cause-analysis-tools/overview/pareto.html.

Associates in Process Improvement (API). (2017). *Associates in process improvement home*. Retrieved from http://www.apiweb.org.

Bialek, R., Duffy, G. L., & Moran, J. W. (2009). *The public health quality improvement handbook*. Milwaukee, WI: ASQ Quality Press.

Center for Medicare and Medicaid Services (CMS). (March 2009). *HCAHPS fact sheet (CAHPS® Hospital Survey). CMS*. Retrieved from http://www.hcahpsonline.org/files/HCAHPS%20Fact%20Sheet,%20revised1,%203-31-09.pdf.

Centers for Medicare and Medicaid Services. (n.d.). *Guidance for performing root cause analysis (RCA) with performance improvement projects (PIPs) failure modes and effects analysis*. Retrieved from https://www.cms.gov/medicare/provider-enrollment-and-certification/qapi/downloads/guidanceforrca.pdf.

Cordon, C. P. (2013). System theories: An overview of various system theories and its application in healthcare. *American Journal of Systems Science*, *21*, 13–22. doi:10.5923/j.ajss.20130201.03.

Fatima, A. (February 28, 2015). *How has the root cause analysis evolved since inception? Bright Hub Project Management*. Retrieved from http://www.brighthubpm.com/risk-management/123244-how-has-the-root-cause-analysis-evolved-since-inception/.

Groene, O., Kringos, D., & Sunol, R. (2014). *Seven ways to improve quality and safety in hospitals. An evidence-based guide. DUQuE Collaboration*. Retrieved from http://www.duque.eu/uploads/DUQuE_Seven_Ways_To_Improve_Quality_And_Safety_2014.pdf.

Institute for Healthcare Improvement (IHI). (2017a). *Quality improvement essentials toolkit*. Cambridge, MA: Institute for Healthcare Improvement. Retrieved from http://www.ihi.org/resources/Pages/Tools/Quality-Improvement-Essentials-Toolkit.aspx.

Institute for Healthcare Improvement (IHI). (2017b). *Science of improvement: How to improve*. Cambridge, MA: Institute for Healthcare Improvement. Retrieved from http://www.ihi.org/resources/Pages/HowtoImprove/ScienceofImprovementHowtoImprove.aspx.

Institute for Healthcare Improvement (IHI). (2017c). *QI essentials toolkit: Failure modes and effects analysis (FMEA) tool*. Cambridge, MA: Institute for Healthcare Improvement. Retrieved from http://www.ihi.org/resources/Pages/Tools/FailureModesandEffectsAnalysisTool.aspx.

Institute for Healthcare Improvement (IHI). (2017d). *QI essentials toolkit: Histogram*. Cambridge, MA: Institute for Healthcare Improvement. Retrieved from http://www.ihi.org/resources/Pages/Tools/Histogram.aspx.

iSixSigma. (2017a). *DMAIC versus DMADV*. Retrieved from https://www.isixsigma.com/new-to-six-sigma/design-for-six-sigma-dfss/dmaic-versus-dmadv/.

iSixSigma. (2017b). *What is six sigma?* Retrieved from https://www.isixsigma.com/new-to-six-sigma/getting-started/what-six-sigma/.

Langley, J. G., Nolan, K. M., Nolan, T. W., Norman, C. L., & Provost, L. P. (2009). *The improvement guide: A practical approach to enhancing organizational performance* (2nd ed.). San Francisco: Jossey-Bass.

Leapfrog Group. (n.d.). *About us: Raising the bar for safer health care.* Retrieved from http://www.leapfroggroup.org/about.

Levinson, W. A., & Rerick, R. A. (2002). *Lean enterprise: A synergistic approach to minimizing waste.* Milwaukee: ASQ Quality Press, xiii-xiv, 38.

Martin, J. R. (n.d.). *Deming's theory of profound knowledge. Management and Accounting Web.* Retrieved from http://maaw.info/DemingExhibit.htm.

Montalvo, I. (September 30, 2007). The national database of nursing quality Indicators™ (NDNQI®) OJIN. *The Online Journal of Issues in Nursing, 12*, 3. doi:10.3912/OJIN.Vol12No03Man02.

National Health Service Institute for Innovation and Improvement. (2011). *Extracts from an improvement framework for commissioners.* Retrieved from http://webarchive.nationalarchives.gov.uk.

QSEN Institute. (2017). *QSEN competencies.* Retrieved from http://qsen.org/competencies/pre-licensure-ksas/#quality_improvement.

Quality-One International. (2015). *5 why & 5 how: Root cause analysis.* Retrieved from https://quality-one.com/5-why-5-how/.

The Joint Commission. (2017). *Performance measures.* Retrieved from https://www.jointcommission.org/performance_measurement.aspx.

The National Learning Consortium (NLC). (2013). *Continuous quality improvement (CQI) strategies to optimize your practice.* Health Information Technology Research Center (HITRC). Retrieved from https://www.healthit.gov/sites/default/files/tools/nlc_continuousqualityimprovementprimer.pdf.

The W. Edwards Deming Institute. (2017a). *The Deming philosophy.* Retrieved from https://deming.org/deming/the-deming-philosophy.

U. S. Department of Health and Human Services Health Resources and Services Administration (HRSA). (2011a). *Quality improvement.* Retrieved from https://www.hrsa.gov/quality/toolbox/508pdfs/qualityimprovement.pdf.

U. S. Department of Health and Human Services Health Resources and Services Administration (HRSA). (2011b). *Developing & implementing a QI plan.* Retrieved from https://www.hrsa.gov/quality/toolbox/508pdfs/qualityimprovement.pdf.

Von Bertalanffy, L. (1968). *General system theory.* New York, NY: George Braziller.

Wagner, E. H., Coleman, K., Reid, R. J., Phillips, K., Abrams, M. K., & Sugarman, J. R. (June 2012). The changes involved in patient centered medical home transformation. *Primary Care, 39*(2), 241–259.

Resources

Health Resources and Services Administration (HRSA) Quality Toolbox. Retrieved from https://www.hrsa.gov/quality/toolbox.

Hughes, R. G. (April 2008). Chapter 44: Tools and strategies for quality improvement and patient safety. In: Hughes R. G. (Ed.), *Patient safety and quality: An evidence-based handbook for nurses.* Rockville, MD: Agency for Healthcare Research and Quality (US). Retrieved from https://www.ncbi.nlm.nih.gov/books/NBK2682.

Institute for Healthcare Improvement Tools. Retrieved from http://www.ihi.org/resources/Pages/Tools/default.aspx.

The W. Edwards Deming Institute. (2017b). *Dr. Deming's 14 points for management.* Retrieved from https://deming.org/explore/fourteen-points.

CHAPTER

3

Nursing Research and Evidence-Based Practice

Al Rundio

This chapter will review:

NURSING RESEARCH

NURSING THEORY

EVIDENCE-BASED PRACTICE

SAMPLE EVIDENCE-BASED PRACTICE PROJECT

Nursing research and evidence-based practice (EBP) has become much more critical as care advances in the 21st century.

This chapter begins with an overview of nursing research and the research process. Following this, information on EBP is discussed. The chapter ends with examples of EBP projects.

Epistemology is the study of knowledge acquisition. When we refer to nursing epistemology, we are generally concerned with knowledge acquisition that improves one's nursing practice. For the sake of this chapter, nursing practice has 4 major areas: clinical practice, administrative practice, education practice, and research practice.

The primary difference between research and EBP is that research poses a question and following exploration answers the question. New knowledge development is the end result. EBP, on the other hand, uses the evidence from primary research and is applied in the clinical setting to see whether improved care occurs.

All research begins with a question.

After the question has been posed, a search of the relevant research literature needs to be conducted. A question commonly raised is what time frame does one go back in the literature? There are differing perspectives on this question; generally, no more than 5 years. One has to consider that, for a study to be published, it usually takes 2 years from submission to the actual publication. (This varies by journal.) What also needs to be considered is the nature of the study. For example, my dissertation was on infection control and I did go back to a seminal study that was conducted in the 1800s because it had relevance to basic hygiene in infection control. I like to look at the 5 years as not a hard-and-fast rule but as a general guideline.

Often the literature search leads to refinement or a restating of the research question. It also provides ideas for the research methodology. I know from experience that if I were comparing injection techniques to measure pain and erythema, I probably would make a comparison on 2 like group of patients. After review of a research article, I could see that there are differences in each group no matter how much alike the groups are. What about skin color? What about pain perception? I then decide from my literature search and review that I will compare both injection techniques on the same patient, which will then allow me to accurately assess erythema and pain in the same patient, which will render more relevant and accurate data.

The steps in the literature search are the following:

Step 1	Determine the concept, issue, topic, or problem that is being explored.
Step 2	Identify key variables and terms.
Step 3	Conduct a computer search for relevant articles.
Step 4	Weed our irrelevant sources that do not address the areas of interest.
Step 5	Organize the relevant sources of information.
Step 6	Retrieve the relevant sources either electronically or in hard copy.
Step 7	Conduct a preliminary reading and further weed out irrelevant sources of information.
Step 8	Critique each source.
Step 9	Summarize each source.
Step 10	Synthesize your findings.

Nursing research is either inductive or deductive.

Inductive implies from specific to broad or from within. One starts with the details of the lived experience and moves toward a general picture. This best describes qualitative research, which uses an inductive approach to the phenomenon being studied.

Deductive research implies from abroad to specific or from without. It is observer detailed. Quantitative research uses this approach wherein the researcher is an observer and not a participant. Quantitative research studies always begin with some theoretical framework. That framework does not need to be a nursing theory. For example, if a researcher were conducting a study on hypertension, the theory of primary hypertension could be used.

RESEARCH CATEGORIES

Basic research describes an exploratory study to explain some phenomenon. Applied research implies an intervention study based on what we learned in the basic study. A case study can be the examination of one or many cases. An example is studying cases of patients with dementia.

Descriptive exploratory research explores and describes some phenomenon. For example, assessing how women feel about body image and middle age. Most researchers have a research trajectory, that is, one study leads to many studies. Often there are more questions raised at the completion of a study than at the beginning, which leads to further studies in that particular field.

Experimental design centers on cause and effect. At a minimum there is one control group and one experimental group. The experimental group gets the intervention, whereas the control group does not. Both groups are evaluated. An example is a pharmaceutical firm that develops a new medication to lower blood pressure. The experimental group would get the intervention of the new medication, whereas the control group would get a placebo and not the intervention. Both groups would have their blood pressure taken at intervals defined by the researcher. The purpose of the research study would be to demonstrate if the new medication indeed lowers blood pressure.

Field research is where a researcher often conducts research in a specific field. For example, nurse researchers may study phenomena in a critical care unit, their field of study.

Historical research examines historical phenomena. One example is the Florence Nightingale Museum in London, England.

Laboratory research is where researchers conduct research. Some nurses achieve higher degrees in pathophysiology, experimentation on mice may be their laboratory. A nurse research who examines education may use a simulation classroom as the laboratory. Laboratory research depends on what type of research the individual does.

Longitudinal research is conducted over a long period. One of the best examples is the Framingham heart study, which studied men with heart disease beginning in 1948 and continues to this day. Certain guidelines today are based on the results from the Framingham study. Examples are lowering the blood pressure, vigorous exercise, and decreasing the cholesterol levels. Another example is the nurse's health study, which is ongoing and examines nurses and health similar to the Framingham study. The Framingham heart study is a great example of how many studies in the past were strictly done with men as the population. There are gender differences when it comes to health and illness, and today many studies incorporate both men and women.

QUALITATIVE RESEARCH STUDIES

Phenomenology is the study of the lived experience. An example is one nurse researcher understanding how a family member could make a do not resuscitate decision on their loved one at a difficult time. This researcher examined 5 such patient families. There were 9 open-ended questions. The family's answers were audiotaped. The audiotapes were transcribed verbatim, and a thematic analysis was completed.

Ethnography examines culture. Many nurse researchers in the past got doctorates in education or anthropology. Ethnography is the study of a culture. An example is examining health practices of Russian immigrants in a major city. One of the best ethnographies and the first ethnography to examine nursing as a culture was completed by Dr. Zane Robinson Wolf from La Salle University in Philadelphia, Pennsylvania. She examined nursing as a culture. She discovered that nursing does many rituals that are not necessarily bad and that these rituals are part of the culture of nursing. Her doctoral dissertation was published by the University of Pennsylvania Press and is titled *Nursing Rituals: The Scared and the Profane.*

Grounded theory is when a qualitative study leads to a new theory. An example is Jean Watson's theory of caring. Another example is the theory of nursing intuition.

Focus groups are a form of phenomenology in which instead of interviewing individuals one interviews a group. This has been used successfully both in clinical research and for market research. Let us view 2 examples. A colleague of mine had a research question that evolved from our work in a correctional health facility as nurse practitioners. The question was why did inmates not always receive their HIV antiviral medication on time? We conducted 2 focus groups of nursing staff and asked 9 open-ended questions. We conducted a thematic analysis on the data with the themes that emerged. We discovered that in correctional health facilities safety took precedence over medicine and nursing. For example, if there was a safety threat, the facility was placed on lockdown and no one would receive medication. There were other reasons as to why medications were not received on time. We learned that the correctional health facility as a place to practice was very different from many other health care organizations. An example of market research is that a hospital wanted to assess market penetration and how consumers felt about their services in a specific geographic region. Two focus groups were conducted with established age and educational parameters. A facilitator was hired for the research. Open-ended questions about health care in the area were presented to the focus group, and a thematic analysis was conducted on the data. The health facility learned information that would benefit them in future planning.

The other categories of qualitative studies have been described previously. They include case studies, descriptive exploratory research, and historical research.

EVALUATION RESEARCH

Evaluation research is a form of research that evaluates a process such as a quality improvement program or a graduate nursing course. There are 2 generic types of evaluation research. The first type, called summative, evaluates a program at the completion of the program. Usually this is a one-time evaluation method. The second type, termed formative, evaluates the process of the program implementation at intervals. For example, a nursing professor teaching a graduate nursing course may conduct an evaluation every other week so that the course can be improved as the course progresses or new topics can be added based on students' participation in the evaluation. Some programs lend themselves well to formative evaluation; other programs are better served by summative evaluation.

RESEARCH TERMS

Quantitative research = numbers.

Qualitative research = words.

Population—The group or sample that is selected to be studied. For statistical purposes, this is usually written as an "n."

Target population—The individuals or things that meet the criteria of interest to the investigator. Sample population—a mini version of the target population, those individuals who meet the criteria of the target population and are available to be in this study.

Validity—This addresses the degree to which an instrument actually measures what it is intended to measure, whether it appropriately assesses the characteristic or construct it is intended to measure, and whether an instrument really measures what it sets out to measure or, instead, measures some other related variable (Polit & Beck, 2017).

Reliability—This refers to the degree of consistency with which an instrument measures whatever it measures. It maximizes the true component of a score and minimizes the error component. It is equated with stability, consistency, and dependability and is sample specific. Reliability is not an enduring property of an instrument. Of the 2 most important concepts of reliability and validity, a test instrument must have validity.

Most instruments are not perfect, and their reliability is expressed as a coefficient number, with 1.00 equaling 100%. The correlation coefficient equal to or greater than .80 is considered an acceptable level of reliability.

TYPES OF SAMPLES

Random sampling—This is a method whereby all members of the population have an equal chance of being selected in the sample population. This avoids research bias.

Convenience sampling—Here the sample is acquired by selecting those participants who are readily available, for example, staff nurses who attend an in-service education program. Convenience sampling can also be referred to as accidental sampling, those people in the right place at the right time.

Purposive sampling—Here the researcher establishes certain criteria, and the subjects are then selected according to the predetermined criteria. For example, if the researcher was examining identical twins, then the sample selected had to be identical twins.

Quota sampling—This allows a maximum number of participants. Many researchers do a power analysis, which determines how powerful their statistics are and predicts the number of participants needed to be in the study.

Snowball sampling—Here a sample population recruits other subjects. One example is a study examining health promotion habits in individuals who have opioid substance use disorders. The researcher seeks individuals who were opioid substance use abusers. The individuals in the sample population could then assist in getting more opioid substance abusers to participate in the study. This can contribute to research bias; however, it is quite useful for difficult-to-obtain sample populations.

EXPERIMENTAL RESEARCH: THE TRUE EXPERIMENT

In the history of the philosophy of science, logical positivists viewed only experimental research designs as true research. Of course, that has changed over the years as we now realize the value of qualitative studies as well as mixed methods research. This section focuses on experimental research or what is termed the true experiment.

There are some factors that separate experimental research from other types of design. There must be a true random sample, that is, everyone in the population has a chance of being selected for that sample. There is more than one group of participants, at a minimum one experimental group and one control group. There is an independent variable, which is manipulated by the researcher, and a dependent variable, which is the outcome variable. For example, when a pharmaceutical firm makes a new medication to lower blood pressure, the new medication will be given to the experimental group and not the control group. The outcome variable or what we term the dependent variable will be the measurement of blood pressure.

In the experimental design the researcher creates a research hypothesis, that is, an educated guess. Hypotheses are tested but not proved, rather they can suggest causation based on inferential statistical analysis. Some researchers begin with the null hypothesis, which states that there is no difference between groups as a result of an intervention in the experimental group. Often the researcher really wants to reject the null hypothesis and accept the alternate hypothesis. The alternate hypothesis states that there is a difference between the 2 groups. Here is an example of the null hypothesis based on our new medication to lower blood pressure. The null hypothesis states that the experimental group when exposed to a new medication to lower blood pressure will have blood pressure readings no different from those of the control group that is not exposed to this or any other intervention. The alternate hypothesis states that the experimental group when exposed to a new medication to lower blood pressure will have blood pressure readings significantly different from those of the control group that is not exposed to new medication or any other intervention.

Often in experimental designs participants in both groups are given a pretest and a posttest. The difference is that the experimental group gets an intervention, whereas the control group does not. The differences between those test scores are compared, and that is how one can conclude significance based on the statistical analyses.

Experimental Design	Pretest	Intervention	Posttest
Experimental group	X	X	X
Control group	X	–	X

DATA SETS

To better understand how to proceed with statistics one must understand data sets. There are 4 primary data sets.

Nominal data—Examples of this are gender, race, and religion. These concepts are representated by some numerical value. The computer uses binary codes. For example, let us look at religion. A researcher may be evaluating health care practices in patients with different religions. A numeric value of 1 may be assigned to Jewish faith, 2 to Protestant faith, 3 to Catholic religion, and so on. This does not mean that Catholics are 3; it just means that 3 represents Catholicism in our study.

Ordinal data—These are data that can be placed in a range one more or less than another, but there is no measurable distance between the data. The best example of this is a pain scale in which patients rate their pain from 0 to 10, zero being no pain and 10 being the greatest amount of pain.

Interval data—These are data that can be placed into a range with a set interval, that is, a set distance from the next point. Examples of this are age and mile markers on a major highway. For example, if I am 50 years old, then I am 5 years older than someone aged 45 years. If I start at mile marker zero on a major highway and travel 20 miles, then I have a measurable distance of 20 miles. Interval data can be both positive and negative numbers. One of the best examples of interval data is a thermometer. Some geographic regions reach below subzero temperatures each winter.

Ratio data—These data have an absolute zero point. One of the best examples is the measurement of weight, as you cannot weigh less than zero. Ratios are also expressed as 3:1, 4:2, etc.

TEST TIP

A good way to remember the types of data sets is to think about a nice wine, such as pinot noir. Think of the word <u>**NOIR**</u>, which stands for **(N)** nominal, **(O)** ordinal, **(I)** interval, and **(R)** ratio data.

MEASURES OF CENTRAL TENDENCY

The mean is the arithmetic average; total the scores of the sample population, then divide by the number of participants in the sample population to arrive at the mean score. The median is the central point; half of the scores fall above the midpoint and half of the scores fall below. The mode is the most frequently occurring number or score.

The purpose of central tendencies is to isolate one response that is representative of the entire sample. In some cases the mean, median, and mode may be identical to each other.

BELL-SHAPED CURVE

Gaussian curve charts—The bell-shaped curve shows frequency distributions.

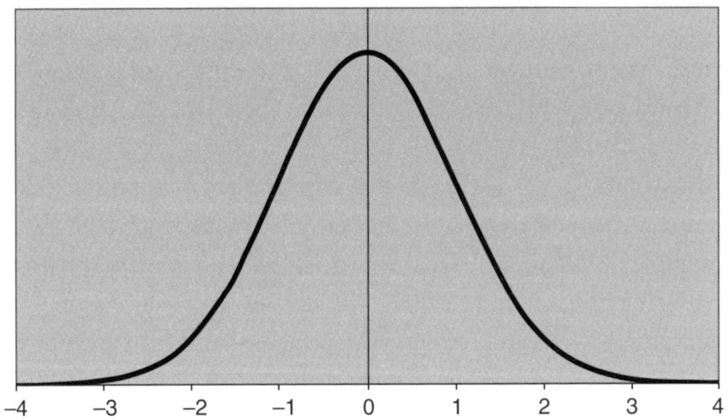

STANDARD DEVIATION

Standard deviation is a measurement of the extent to which samples are away from the center (mean). Different samples have different means.

LEVEL OF SIGNIFICANCE

Think back to your very first statistics course in college. What did your professor do on the first day? I attended a school in South Jersey near Atlantic City, one of the casino capitals of the world. My professor started the first statistics class by bringing 2 red dice to class. He rolled the **dice** until he got 6's on. The question to the class was what is the probability that I could roll 2 dice with 6's on it again? I was not sure what he was talking about, but now I understand it much better. He was demonstrating that, in research, results can happen by chance alone. Unless the dice were rigged in some way so that with each roll two sixes would come up then the probability would be predictable. This is not the case in research studies as results can occur by chance alone.

The level of significance refers to getting the same result by chance alone. There is never a perfect research study. Therefore, there is never a 100% time that a researcher can predict what will happen. Generally 2 levels of significance are used by researchers. The first level is the 95% level. This implies that 95% of the time the results of the intervention occurred because of the intervention and 5% of the time it could happen by chance alone. The other level of significance used by researchers is the 99% level. This implies that there is 1 of 100 times that the results could occur by chance alone. The other 99 times the result occurred from the intervention.

It is critical to understand the concepts of level of significance when we are dealing with experimental designs. As you recall, the purpose of an experimental design is to demonstrate causation, that is, that the result was because of the intervention.

CLINICAL SIGNIFICANCE

Clinical significance is an interesting concept to discuss. Findings can have statistical significance but not clinical significance or vice versa. As nursing is a practice discipline, the concept of clinical significance is important. Clinical significance relates to the practical importance of the findings. There is really no common agreement in nursing about how to judge clinical significance. Is it the effect size? Is there a difference sufficiently important to warrant changing the patient's care? This then is up to the researcher to determine if clinical significance exists.

TYPE I AND TYPE II ERRORS

With the confidence intervals that were described, what one is really doing is testing the null hypothesis and the alternate hypothesis.

An error can occur based on the inferential statistics that the researcher does in either rejecting or accepting the null hypothesis. In order for there to be significance where the null hypothesis is rejected, the researcher must have a key value equal to or less than 0.05 or equal to or less than 0.01, depending on which confidence interval the researcher selected. If the calculated inferential statistic is greater than those numbers, then the person would accept the null hypothesis, as there is no difference, and the interpretation would be that the intervention did not cause the result. If the calculated inferential statistic is less than those numbers, then the researcher would reject the null hypothesis, and the interpretation here is that the intervention caused the results.

Type I Error

A type I error results when the data analysis indicates that the null hypothesis should be rejected; it is committed if in reality the null hypothesis is true. If the null hypothesis is false, then a correct decision was made.

Type II Error

A type II error results when the data analysis indicates that results are not significant and the null hypothesis is accepted. In reality the null hypothesis is true, so a correct decision has been made. If in reality the null hypothesis is false and the researcher should have rejected the null hypothesis but he or she did not, then a type II error was committed.

The following table demonstrates type I and II errors:

Data Analysis Indicates	In Reality Null Hypothesis Is True	In Reality Null Hypothesis Is False
Results are significant and null hypothesis is rejected	Type I error	Correct decision (power)
Results are not significant and null hypothesis is accepted	Correct decision	Type II error

STATISTICAL TEST MEASURES

There are 2 major types of statistics.

Descriptive statistics—These statistics describe the data through the use of charts, tables, and graphs. They can be used both in quantitative and qualitative research studies. Even though qualitative studies are generally words, some data can be displayed in a table, chart, or graph. For example, a colleague of mine surveyed patients in an obstetric clinic about their knowledge of HIV transmission. She had a very large sample for a qualitative study of 105 participants. These participants consented to HIV testing before the study. A total of 103 of the participants were HIV negative, 1 was HIV positive, and 1 was HIV in determinant. She could certainly explain these data through the use of descriptive statistics.

Inferential statistics—To utilize these statistics in a research study; the researcher must use statistical testing measures on data sets. To perform these statistics the research study must have quantitative data. There are 2 broad classifications of inferential statistics.

Parametric—Parametric statistics must have interval or ratio data. Logical positivists would consider this true science.

Nonparametric—Nonparametric statistics uses nominal or ordinal data. There are inferential statistics for both types of data. One should refer to a nursing research text for a description of all types of inferential statistics and the data that is required.

There are many different types of inferential statistics. The following describes the most common ones that are utilized.

T-test for independent samples—This tests the difference between the means of 2 independent groups.

T-test for dependent paired samples—This tests the difference between the means of 2 related groups of sets of scores.

ANOVA—This tests the difference among the means of 3 or more independent groups or more than one independent variable.

Chi square—This tests the difference in proportions in 2 or more groups.

Fisher's Exact—This tests the difference in proportions in a 2 × 2 contingency table in which the sample size is less than 30.

Pearson product moment correlation—This tests that a correlation is different from zero (that a relationship exists).

Spearman's rho—This tests that a correlation is different from zero (that a relationship exists).

MORE ON QUALITATIVE RESEARCH

As previously discussed, qualitative research views the lived experience. It is action oriented and is words rather than numbers. Descriptive statistics can be used to display certain data elements, such as the composition of the sample population. It is research generally conducted through open-ended questions, audiotapes, art, literature, and experience. The researcher completes thematic analysis where concepts and themes are identified.

MIXED METHODS RESEARCH

Mixed methods research has really become one of the types of research that is used the most. In mixed methods the researcher incorporates both quantitative and qualitative research designs. Excellent data can be obtained from mixed methods research. The results are quite thorough because of both the quantitative and qualitative approach to the research study.

ETHICAL ISSUES IN RESEARCH

A great topic to have test questions on would be ethical issues in research. This goes back to the Nuremberg trials of Nazi Germany, which set the tone for the conduct of future research on human subjects. The United States certainly has had unethical research. One should read about the Tuskegee Syphilis Trial in Alabama. The U.S. Department of Health and Human Services has guidelines for the conduct of research on human subjects in the United States.

Research consent—The research consent must be informed, detailed in layman's terms at the reading level that is appropriate for the subjects. Usually this reading level is no higher than the sixth grade. The consent must state that subjects can withdraw from the research program at any time without being penalized regardless of whether they are being paid to be in the study or not (Polit & Beck, 2017).

Research ascent—Minors sign a research ascent, which is permission for the research to occur. This is for minors of age who can understand what is happening with the research.

Institutional review board (IRB)—IRB is critical to the protection of human subjects. Its major charge is to protect human subjects during the research process. It should be composed of 50% of members who have no affiliation with the facility where the research is being conducted and going for IRB approval. This is so that there is an objective view to the research process and the protection of human subjects. IRBs review in cycles, and this varies according to the type of institution. For example, a large academic health science center most likely has IRB reviews and meetings every other week, whereas a small community hospital may have its IRB meet on a quarterly basis.

Expedited review—Expedited review occurs for studies that do not involve invasive interventions on patients. For example, projects that center more on quality improvement would be reviewed by the IRB chair for approval and then he/she would present it at the next IRB meeting.

Central IRB—When multisite studies are conducted, the study may be reviewed first by a central IRB, which is an IRB separate from any of the institutions involved in the study. This provides a totally objective review. The study will still need to be approved by each institution, but once central IRB approval has been obtained the approval process is usually much quicker at the individual institution.

Once approval is obtained from the IRB and the study commences, any time an untoward outcome occurs it must be reported promptly to the IRB. When the study is completed, a summary of the results must be sent to the IRB so that the study can be officially closed down. To submit to the IRB most institutions require that one has either current National Institutes of Health training or CITI training. One Web site that you may want to visit is the IRB computer-based training from the National Institutes of Health. This is free of charge, and anyone can take this program. This is also a great way to study for research questions on the nursing certification examination.

RESEARCH IDEAS

To conclude this section on research, let us examine some potential research ideas. What phenomenon needs investigation at your institution? What question is present in your practice that requires answers? What about replication research?

Examples

If you practice in addictions nursing, what about counseling therapies and their effectiveness? What about relapse prevention strategies for clients? What about relapse pharmacology and its effectiveness? If you are an advanced practice nurse (APN), what is the role of the APN on the outcome of patient care? For any type of practice what is learner readiness in clients? For nurse executives what are the staffing patterns in the relationship to patient care and outcomes? Are 12-hour shifts the best for safety and quality? What about 10-hour shifts or 8-hour shifts?

And certainly the myriad of clinical problems and interventions that we do as nurses every day in practice.

EVIDENCE-BASED PRACTICE

Thomas Kuhn was a wonderful philosopher. In his classic book published in 1970 titled *The Nature Scientific of Revolutions*, Kuhn describes and contrasts normal science to that of a paradigm. According to Kuhn, normal science involves continuing research that concerns a particular field of study. A paradigm is a working model. Scientific revolutions result when there is a major paradigm shift. A relevant example is HIV disease. Before the virus was discovered, the working knowledge that we had focused on prevention through sexual transmission. Not that that is still not important, but when the virus was discovered a new paradigm shift occurred. Research could now focus on antiretroviral and other therapies to stop the progression of HIV disease. Another example is chaos theory. Chaos theory refutes classic physics theory. In physics, everything was thought to be regular and predictable. Then through the use of computer modeling a new theory was developed called chaos, which is characterized by randomness, irregularity, and unpredictability.

This section began with Kuhn because EBP is a major paradigm shift in how one practices today. EBP is truly transforming health care and improving patient care outcomes.

What then is the difference between primary research and EBP? The following chart describes these differences.

Primary Research	**Evidence-Based Practice**
Posing a question	Posing a clinically relevant question
Searching the literature	Searching the literature for evidence
Reviewing the literature	Critically appraising the evidence
Theory	Frameworks
Methodology	PICOT format
Statistics/words	Outcomes
Generation of new knowledge	Knowledge translation

A Little About Magnet Status

There is no question that the Magnet Recognition Program and other initiatives have promoted research and EBP; however, if nursing is really an art and a science, then practice needs to be rooted in research and research evidence. Both the art and the science need exploration, validation, and testing.

According to Sackett, Straus, Richardson, Rosenberg, and Haynes (2000) as cited in Melnyk and Fineout-Overholt (2014), EBP is the conscientious use of current best evidence in making decisions about patient care.

Let us review the following question. From your clinical assessment you have to make a decision on a treatment for a patient. When you search the literature, there are only 2 pieces of evidence that answers the question. What should you do? There are a variety of things that one could do. You could review the 2 pieces of evidence to see which one rated higher on the critical appraisal scale. You could call colleagues to see what they have done with the same situation in the past. You would also have to look at fiscal resources. If the intervention involves a high price tag, does your institution have the resources to fund this? Certainly more research evidence is warranted, but there is no time to do this when you need to make such a clinical decision.

The question that needs to be raised then is "Is it really evidence-based practice or are we really talking about evidence-based decision-making?" There are many interventions that we do that are not yet based on evidence but certainly on one's clinical expertise and experience. So at times we make decisions for patient care that are really based on whatever evidence is available to us, and at times, that may not be a lot of research evidence.

EBP involves completing a systematic search for the evidence. Then one critically appraises the most relevant evidence that attempts to answer a burning clinical question. There are a variety of critical appraisal tools available. It also involves one's own clinical expertise and experience as well as patient's preferences and values. Considering a patient's preferences and values is crucial. Patients may be told to take a medication to lower cholesterol but they may not want to take the medication. They may try herbal supplements. Even though the evidence may suggest that the patient should be on the cholesterol-lowering medication, the patient may elect not to do so.

According to Melnyk and Fineout-Overholt (2014), the 6 steps of EBP are the following:

Step 0	Create a spirit of inquiry
Step 1	The need for information that is placed into a clinically relevant, answerable question
Step 2	Systematic retrieval of the best evidence that is available
Step 3	Critical appraisal of evidence for validity and clinical relevance
Step 4	Application of critically appraised evidence in clinical practice
Step 5	Evaluation of outcomes

Clinical Judgment and Evidence-Based Practice

Decision-making/problem-solving: incorporates skills of engaged practical reasoning, that is, recognition of a pattern.

Clinical judgment: understanding about a patient's needs, concerns, or health problems, followed by the decision to act or not to act, to use or modify standard approaches as deemed appropriate by the patient's clinical response.

Clinical reasoning: a thinking process by which clinicians make their judgments and includes the process of generating alternatives and weighing the risk against the evidence in choosing the correct course of action.

Why Evidence-Based Practice?

EBP is done to achieve the best patient outcomes, reduce health care costs, reduce geographic variations in the care rendered, and promote and retain health care workers. In spite of these many benefits, familiarity and implementation of EBP remains low. Approximately 75% of what we do today in health care is based on current evidence. It generally takes 13 to 17 years to take the evidence and actually implement it in practice. One way to improve EBP is through much earlier implementation of the evidence.

Initiatives to Advance Evidence-Based Practice

The following are initiatives to advance EBP:

- Institute of Medicine's Roundtable on Evidence-Based Medicine
- United States Preventive Services Task Force (USPSTF)
- Agency for Healthcare Research and Quality (AHRQ)
- National Consortium for the Advancement of Pediatric and Adolescent Evidence-Based Practice (NCPAEP)
- Magnet Recognition Program by the American Nurses Credentialing Center (ANCC)

EBP generally follows the **PICOT** framework. This framework is an excellent way in which to put the clinical question into a usable format.

P = the patient population or problem of interest
I = the intervention or issue of interest
C = a comparative intervention or group
O = outcome
T = the time frame in which the intervention will be evaluated

SAMPLE EVIDENCE RATING SCALE

Level 1: Systematic reviews or meta-analyses of rigorous controlled clinical trials
Level 2: Rigorous controlled clinical trials
Level 3: Controlled trials without randomization
Level 4: Case-control and cohort studies
Level 5: Systematic reviews of descriptive and qualitative studies
Level 6: Single descriptive or qualitative studies
Level 7: Opinion of authorities and/or reports of expert committees

SAMPLE MODIFIED EVIDENCE RATING SCALE

Level I (strong)—Experimental design (randomized controlled trial) or a meta-analysis of randomized controlled trials (rigorously controlled clinical trial)

Level II—Quasi-experimental designs

Level III—Nonexperimental studies; qualitative study; a metasynthesis of qualitative studies

Level IV—Clinical expertise

Level V—Patient preferences and values

When critically appraising the evidence, pay attention to validity, reliability, and applicability. The goal of EBP is to integrate the best evidence with clinical expertise and patient preferences. This can be termed the implementation step. EBP is not based solely on research and published evidence. It is also based on the patient's history and circumstances. These have a significant bearing on the nurse's choice of an intervention. One also must consider the available resources.

Following implementation it is necessary to evaluate the outcomes of the practice decision. The measurement of outcomes is important to determine and document the impact of the EBP change on health care quality and patient outcomes. It is essential in determining whether the change based on the evidence resulted in the expected outcomes when implemented in the real-world practice setting.

Just as in research, it is important to disseminate the outcomes of the EBP decision. Too often in health care, positive outcomes are not shared with others. The goal is really to improve care for all patients no matter where they are. There are numerous strategies for disseminating and accomplishing the goal. This can be anything from personal communication to publications, poster presentations, white papers, and presentations at conferences.

Barriers to Evidence-Based Practice

There are many barriers to EBP. Some of the major ones are the following:

- Lack of knowledge
- Information overload
- Lack of role models
- Lack of time or money
- Resistance to change
- Misperceptions such as I have to have a doctorate to do EBP

Facilitators of Evidence-Based Practice

- Support from leaders and peers
- Adequate time
- Resources
- Journal clubs
- EBP rounds

A determined effort is often required to address barriers and facilitate the implementation of EBP.

Let us begin where we started from. To do EBP, one must question the clinical practice, be willing to change that practice, and be willing to evaluate the impact. Health care professionals must ask questions about their current practice. Practice problems should be prioritized, for example, what is the most serious, pressing problem? Change requires vision, planning, and persistence.

Cars that are built today are based on research evidence. One example is how the wearing of seat belts has become mandatory in most states. As the manufacturers of our automobiles evaluate evidence and change how a car is built, should we as health providers not be doing the same for our patients? The question is not when or if we should do, the question is why are we not doing it?

SAMPLE EVIDENCE-BASED DNP PROJECT

Chapter 1: Introduction/Background Information

The impetus for this project resulted from several factors affecting advanced nursing practice in the field of addictions.

As an APN certified by the American Nurses Credentialing Center as an Acute Care Nurse Practitioner and an Adult Health Primary Care Nurse Practitioner as well as certified by the International Nurses Society of Addictions as a Certified Addictions Registered Nurse—Advanced Practice and licensed as a Licensed Clinical Alcohol and Drug Counselor by the Board of Marriage and Family Therapy in New Jersey, my primary area of practice for the past 11 years has been the field of addictions.

The role of the APN in the facility that I practice at was conceptualized by myself and happened by circumstance rather than a well-defined plan. The Medical Director of the facility was involved in a serious car accident in 1997, and I received a telephone call both from him and the Director of Nursing requesting that I cover him for a few-day period. Medical rounds had not been made for several days, and several patients needed the required history and physical examination performed as well as all other routine medical orders. I accepted the offer to be of assistance, and what evolved was full implementation of an advanced practice nursing role, thus shifting the facility from a pure medical model of care delivery to that of an advanced practice nursing model with medical oversight. The current Medical Director is extremely supportive of the advanced practice nursing model. Our collaborative role has been to continually improve the facility and the care rendered to our patients with good-quality medical and nursing care.

PICOT

Patient Population. The patient population consists of adult patients between the ages of 18 years and the elderly, although the vast majority of our patients are young adults. These patients are chemically addicted to various substances and are admitted to a residential inpatient treatment facility for detoxification from such substances. A small percentage of the patients are admitted for rehabilitation only, as they have already been detoxified from substances. Detoxification of this latter group of patients resulted by patient self-detoxification or by detoxification at another facility before completing a residential rehabilitation program.

The treatment facility is a for-profit, private residential treatment facility located in southern New Jersey. This treatment facility is licensed by the New Jersey State Department of Health to provide both acute medical detoxification of patients and rehabilitation services. The facility is licensed for 62 inpatient beds. There are 2 primary treatment units at this facility. The adolescent unit is licensed for 42 inpatient beds. Patients admitted to the adolescent unit are between the ages of 13 and 18 years. The adult unit is licensed for 20 inpatient beds. Of the 20 licensed adult beds, 15 are for acute medical detoxification and 5 are for rehabilitation purposes. This treatment facility is accredited by the Joint Commission on Accreditation of Health Care Organizations. This treatment facility also has 3 intensive outpatient treatment programs. One program is housed at the treatment facility. The other 2 treatment programs are housed off-site. One program is located in Ventnor, New Jersey, a border community to Atlantic City. The other outpatient program is located in Manahawkin, another Jersey Shore community in Ocean County, New Jersey. This project focuses only on the adult inpatient population.

Intervention. The role of advanced practice nursing in addictions includes the medical detoxification of patients. Patients, when detoxified from substances, are gradually weaned down on the medication used for acute detoxification. Abrupt withdrawal of a medication could trigger acute withdrawal symptoms in patients, which could be potentially life-threatening in some circumstances.

The advanced practice role includes making daily medical and nursing rounds. Each day either the Medical Director or the APN had to write new orders for detoxification to wean the patient down. For example, if an alcoholic patient was given chlordiazepoxide (Librium) 50 mg every 6 hours for 24 hours, the next day a new order had to be written that lowered the Librium dose, for example, Librium 35 mg every 6 hours for 24 hours. The APN questioned if there was a more efficient manner in which to detoxify patients. The suggestion was to develop medical and nursing protocols for detoxification that would be a standard order set for patients. This was supported by the Director of Nursing at the facility, as she had just had a consultant review the facility for efficiency. His recommendation was also to develop treatment protocols. With the movement toward EBP, the Medical Director fully supported this concept and charged the APN with the development of such protocols. A meeting was conducted with the Medical Director, the Director of Nursing, and the Advanced Practice Nurse. It was decided that the treatment protocols should be evidence based and should incorporate current relapse prevention medications as well as the routine detoxification medications. To date, 10 treatment protocols have been developed and implemented based on the common substances abused by patients who are admitted to this particular treatment facility. Certain abused substances, such as alcohol and opioids, have a few treatment protocols so that correct dosing of detoxification medication can be tailored to patient use and abuse patterns. The common substances abused by the patients include the following:

- Alcohol
- Anabolic steroids
- Anxiolytics (benzodiazepines [BZDs], barbiturates)
- Amphetamines
- Club drugs (Ecstasy, γ-hydroxybutyrate [GHB], Rohypnol)
- Cocaine
- Marijuana (tetrahydrocannabinol)
- Nicotine
- Psychedelics/hallucinogens

Exclusion Criteria

- Pregnant patients
- Patient with gambling addictions
- Patient with sexual addictions
- Adolescent patients (13–17 years of age)

Treatment protocols have been developed for alcohol, BZDs, and opioids. The benefits to the development of such protocols included the following:

1. Standardized written order form that was computer generated
2. Standardized patient care protocol
3. Pharmacologic and other interventions based on current evidence in the field
4. Decrease in variation of both written orders and patient care
5. Measurement and evaluation of treatment interventions
6. Decrease in the time needed to write daily orders
7. Flexibility for change as new evidence is discovered

Comparison Intervention/Status. It was decided to implement all of the protocols at the same time with concurrent evaluation, rather than using a comparative group with a different intervention. It was the overriding feeling that the medical and nursing practitioners would be able to assess if the treatment protocols were more effective than daily handwritten orders. This would be assessed primarily through patient response, nursing input and feedback, and formal evaluation.

Outcome. Outcome evaluation will consist of direct observation and qualitative evaluation with use of a focus group of nurses.

I. Outcome evaluation
  A. Quantitative and qualitative evaluation with defined indicators 3 months after implementation of project
    1. Direct observation of patients by nursing and medical staffs
      a. Concurrent chart audit with defined indicators
        i. Number of seizures
        ii. Vital signs
        iii. Number of times PRN medications are used (based on Clinical Institute Withdrawal Assessment [CIWA] [alcohol] scale)
        iv. Pain Assessment Scale
        v. Number of times detoxification protocols have to be readjusted
    2. Qualitative focus group of nursing staff with open-ended interview questions

Chapter 2: Conceptual Framework

Addiction fits a biopsychosocial/spiritual disease model. According to Ott, Tarter, and Ammerman (1999) "it is difficult to search for single determining factors in a complex world where the individual human being is one biopsychosocial system" (p. 175). Current research in the field has reinforced the biological components to this disease process. For several years now, health practitioners have been aware that addiction is a "real" disease. Addicts do not elect to become addicted. With the advent of positive emission tomography scanning, brain chemistry and neurochemical transmitter release have been studied. Many receptor sites in the primitive brain area called the ventral trigeminal area have been identified, for example, opium receptors, cocaine receptors, and alcohol receptors. Some theories on addiction are that clients may have damaged receptor sites or genetic mutations that affect neurochemical release and saturation of receptor sites. Certainly, the psychology of the individual as well as the sociologic manifestations also contributes to addiction. Spirituality has brought many individuals to recovery. It is one of the founding philosophies of 12-step programs. From my experience from doing several history and physical examinations over the years, I have observed many clients who do not relate to any spiritual entity when they are addicted.

The best way to view addictions is to view it as a chronic disease process. This model certainly fits addictions. Just as a diabetic may have high blood glucose level after ingesting a large piece of cake, addicts also can relapse and turn back to substance use and abuse. Providers need to be understanding of patients who relapse, as any chronic disorder can have reoccurrences. Clinicians should not judge individuals who relapse, but rather support their recovery until it is permanent.

One of the primary goals of treatment is to address the components of this model. The biological aspect of addictions is accomplished through pharmacology both for detoxification and relapse prevention. The psychological component is addressed through psychiatric evaluation of the client, as many clients have an underlying psychiatric disorder. The social component is addressed by including the family and significant others (SOs) in the treatment process. The goal of treatment is to get clients to lead an effective life that includes returning to work or finding employment. As with any disease process, family inclusiveness is necessary, as family members can be enablers, which is contradictory to the philosophy of treatment. The spiritual component is addressed through 12-step meetings, such as Alcoholics Anonymous, where an individual having a belief in a "higher power" is one of the founding steps in this process.

This project focused primarily on the biological aspect of this conceptual model. Ten treatment protocols were developed, implemented, and evaluated, which incorporated current evidence on pharmacologic interventions for both detoxification of addicts and pharmacology focused on relapse prevention.

Chapter 3: Review of the Literature

Alcohol

According to Lejoyeux, Solomon, and Ades (1998) and Ott et al. (1999), BZDs are the preferred pharmacologic agents for the treatment of acute alcohol withdrawal states. The authors further state that mild to moderate withdrawal symptoms can be treated with BZDs on an outpatient basis, whereas severe withdrawal states require inpatient admission. Lejoyeux et al. (1998) state that BZDs do not improve abstinence rates and in most circumstances are not indicated for long-term use. A variety of BZDs can be used for successful detoxification. Librium is the gold standard for treatment of alcohol withdrawal states. Lorazepam (Ativan) has also been used with success and is often the preferred treatment in the acute care hospital setting, as Ativan can be administered intravenously as well as orally. One of the problems with use of the BZDs is their long half-life. In some patients with liver failure secondary to cirrhosis and alcoholism, BZDs given orally are not processed quickly enough by the failing liver. Oxazepam (Serax) as an alternative BZD has been found to be more effective in these cases.

Phillips, Haycock, and Boyle (2006) designed a process improvement project that developed an alcohol withdrawal syndrome (AWS) management protocol for the acute care hospital setting. The design of this project included a work team that comprised physicians, pharmacists, and nurses led by a behavioral health clinical nurse specialist. The outcome of this project was the development and integration of a safe and effective treatment protocol that effectively managed AWS. This project was facilitated by collaborative, evidence-based decision-making. The authors addressed 3 key components of care: (1) the identification of high-risk patients, (2) the initiation of prophylactic treatment, and (3) the initiation of effective and timely pharmacologic interventions in an effort to prevent medical complications in AWS that could lead to death. The authors also concluded from their review that BZDs are the mainstay of primary pharmacologic therapy in patients in AWS. Their preferred medication in the acute care setting was diazepam (Valium).

Nimmerrichter, Walter, Gutierrez-Lobos, and Lesch (2002) conducted a double-blind controlled trail of GHB (γ-hydroxybutyrate) and clomethiazole in the treatment of alcohol withdrawal symptoms. The purpose of the study was to assess GHB's efficacy and safety in ameliorating symptoms of alcohol withdrawal. Subjects were randomized to receive either clomethiazole or GHB. One clomethiazole group was established. Two GHB groups were established whereby the dosage of the GHB varied by group. The authors concluded that there was no difference between the 3 treatment groups in the rating of alcohol withdrawal symptoms. There were also no requests for additional medication. After tapering of medication, there was no increase in withdrawal symptoms noted or requests for medication. This indicated that physical tolerance did not develop in any of the groups. The most frequently reported side effect was in the GHB group, which reported transient vertigo after the evening double dosage of medication. GHB used to be sold as a "health tonic" in health food stores until the potential for abuse was discovered. GHB overdose can cause a cessation of respiration, coma, and death. GHB was pulled off of the market a few years ago. As a result of this, GHB is usually not found in treatment protocols for alcohol dependency.

Relapse Prevention

Ott et al. (1999) state that "although the substitution of an abused drug with a safer controlled medication, such as methadone, for the treatment of opioid dependence has been shown to be effective, recent pharmacotherapy developments in alcohol and cocaine dependence focus more on nonsubstitution treatment (e.g. relapse prevention, reduction of craving) with medications that are not themselves habit forming" (p. 303).

Relapse prevention incorporates the use of other types of pharmacologic agents. Disulfiram (Antabuse) has been on the market for several years now. Many clinicians have stopped prescribing this medication secondary to life-threatening reactions, including death in patients who drink alcohol when taking Antabuse. According to Ott et al. (1999), Antabuse may be an effective treatment for cocaine dependency; however, the authors caution that further research is warranted first.

Streeton and Whelan (2001) conducted a meta-analysis of naltrexone use as a relapse-prevention medication for alcoholism. The authors searched MEDLINE, EMBASE, PsychLIT, and Cochrane Controlled Trials Registry for articles published from 1976 to 2001. Their meta-analysis demonstrated that naltrexone was superior to placebo. Subjects in the naltrexone treatment groups maintained abstinence longer and had fewer episodes of relapse compared with those in the control groups. In 2006 a pharmaceutical firm developed Vivitrol, an injectable form of naltrexone. Vivitrol is administered on a once-monthly basis and is ideal for patients who have elevated liver enzymes, as oral naltrexone is contraindicated in such patients. Vivitrol must be ordered through the pharmaceutical firm that developed the medication and not at a standard retail pharmacy. It is important for clinicians to recognize that pharmacotherapy cannot reverse personal and social disruptions that are experienced by substance abusers, thus the need for psychosocial approaches conjointly with pharmacotherapy (Ott et al., 1999).

Acamprosate (Campral) has also been demonstrated to be an effective relapse prevention medication for alcoholism. Although the exact mechanism of action of Campral is not completely understood, according to Ott et al. (1999) the available evidence suggests that it enhances the function of *N*-methyl-D-aspartate, an amino acid receptor. This medication is currently used in treatment as a relapse prevention medication, as it improves abstinence outcome and diminishes cravings for alcohol. The standard dose of Campral is 666 mg administered 3 times daily orally.

Brown (1973); Liebson, Bigelow, and Flamer (1973); and El-Bassel, Shilling, Turnbull, and Su (1993) estimate that alcohol dependency rates vary from 5% to 49% among participants in methadone maintenance programs. Caputo et al. (2002) evaluated alcohol use in nonalcoholic heroin addicts during the first 4 weeks of a treatment program. The treatment program consisted of either a methadone maintenance program or a non-methadone maintenance program. The authors note that many heroin-dependent clients will begin to abuse alcohol when in treatment. A total of 359 heroin-addicted subjects were enrolled on an outpatient basis. All patients met the Diagnostic and Statistical Manual of Mental Disorders, 4th Edition, criteria. Thirty-two subjects dropped out of the study. The authors noted a significant decrease in the daily alcohol intake in the methadone maintenance program compared with the nonmethadone maintenance program. The authors concluded that the results of the study suggested a possible effect in reducing alcohol consumption by administering methadone on a short-term basis to nonalcoholic heroin-addicted patients.

Opioids

Various pharmacologic agents have been used for the management of withdrawal symptoms secondary to opioid dependency. As opioid withdrawal consists of a constellation of flu-like symptoms, including muscle aches and pains, some pharmacologic measures have included the following: muscle relaxants; methadone; LAAM (l-α-acetylmethadol or levo-methadyl acetate); clonidine; phenobarbital; amantadine (Symmetrel); Librium; nonsteroidal antiinflammatory drugs; and propoxyphene (Darvon). According to Ott et al. (1999), LAAM is a much longer-acting opioid agonist compared with methadone. The half-life of LAAM is estimated to be greater than 100 hours. Having 11 years of experience in addictions nursing, I have never seen LAAM used in practice.

Withdrawal symptoms from opioids are generally not life-threatening. As such, newer agents on the market that contribute to office-based treatment of opioid dependency have been used. According to Fiellin, Rosenheck, and Kosten (2001), the Drug Addiction Treatment Act of 2000 allowed qualifying physicians to prescribe schedule III, IV, and V narcotic medications or combinations of such medications for treating opioid-dependent patients. Buprenorphine (marketed as Subutex and Suboxone) came on the market for such office-based practice. According to Fiellin et al. (2001), buprenorphine has 3 major advantages over other available alternative pharmacologic agents. These advantages are the following: (1) The medication is a partial opioid agonist; thus the associated withdrawal syndrome is milder; (2) the effect of this pharmacologic agent is long-lasting; thus dosing can be limited to 2- to 3-day intervals, reducing associated clinic visits; and (3) buprenorphine can be combined with naloxone, an opioid antagonist that blocks the effect of abuse with another opioid and also allows the medication to be administered sublingually. Ott et al. (1999) state that naloxone does not precipitate withdrawal symptoms in those patients who have been pretreated with buprenorphine. They further state that withdrawal from an 8-mg dose of buprenorphine has milder withdrawal symptoms compared with other agents, and also buprenorphine creates less dependence than other medications, such as methadone. To date, only physicians are approved to administer this medication. According to the Food and Drug Administration, APNs may not prescribe this medication. Some physicians have petitioned the Food and Drug Administration to allow prescribing of this medication by APNs. This is an advanced practice issue confronting APNs in the field of addictions.

Physicians who prescribe this medication must attend an 8-hour course on this pharmacologic agent. Initially the law permitted a physician to have only 30 patients at a time in his or her practice. If the practice had more than one physician, then each physician could have 30 patients in the practice provided that he or she attended the 8-hour program. The law was revised, and physicians are now permitted to have up to 100 patients in their practice who are being prescribed buprenorphine. This medication is highly regulated at this time, and physician offices are subject to surprise inspections by the Drug Enforcement Agency. Fiellin et al. (2001) state that new patient populations have been reached with the advent of buprenorphine.

The primary pharmacologic agent for relapse prevention in opioid-dependent addicts is naltrexone. Research to date has demonstrated that the pharmacologic agent by itself does not contribute to long-term sobriety. Combination therapy with other modalities, such as cognitive behavioral therapy and

12-step meetings, contribute to longer-term sobriety. Carroll et al. (2001) conducted a study in which contingency management (CM), a behavioral therapy intervention, and SO involvement were evaluated as strategies to enhance treatment retention and medication compliance with naltrexone, thus contributing to longer-term sobriety. A total of 127 recently detoxified opioid-dependent patients were randomized to 1 of 3 treatment groups for a 12-week period. The groups included the following: (1) standard naltrexone treatment; (2) naltrexone treatment and CM; and (3) naltrexone treatment, CM, and SO involvement. SO involvement was described as a family member who was invited to participate in up to 6 family counseling sessions. Outcomes focused on retention in treatment, compliance with naltrexone therapy, and the number of urine specimens that were drug free. The group that had the most significant improvement outcomes was the CM group. This group demonstrated treatment retention and a reduction in opioid use. SO involvement did not significantly improve retention, compliance, or outcomes compared with the CM group. SO involvement was associated with improved family functioning. The authors concluded that behavioral therapies, such as CM, are important to improved compliance with pharmacologic interventions. This study supports the notion that pharmacology alone is not sufficient, and as substance abuse is a chronic disease process, various targeted therapies must be used to adequately treat the patient.

Other Abused Substances

The literature is replete with information about other abused substances. For example, to date, there is no relapse prevention medication for cocaine dependency, although clinical trials are currently exploring baclofen use in this population. The vast majority of substances are treated pharmacologically as the patient presents with various symptoms. The majority of these substances, for example, cocaine, amphetamines, club drugs, marijuana (tetrahydrocannabinol), and anabolic steroids, are treated based on patient presenting symptoms. Routine treatment protocols are generally not used in these patient populations.

Summary

Positive emission tomography scanning is leading the way for the clinical trials of many newer and older medications for both treatment as well as relapse prevention in addicted patients. The 2 substances that the literature discusses most frequently is alcoholism and opioid dependency. Relapse pharmacologic agents are now recommended for these 2 substances when they are abused.

Chapter 4: Project Description

Ten detoxification treatment protocols, 3 alcohol, 1 BZD, and 6 opioid, were developed based on current evidence in the field. Different detoxification treatment protocols for alcohol and opioid dependency were developed to be able to curtail pharmacologic dosing with patient use and withdrawal symptom patterns. Detoxification treatment protocols included relapse prevention pharmacology where applicable. All detoxification treatment protocols were developed by an APN at the treatment facility who is currently certified as a Certified Registered Nurse in Addictions Advanced Practice by the International Nurses Society on Addictions. All detoxification treatment protocols were reviewed and approved by the Medical Director at the treatment facility, who is currently board certified in addictions medicine by the American Society of Addictions Medicine and the Executive Committee at the treatment facility (equivalent to IRB approval in other settings—see Appendix A).

Following development of the detoxification treatment protocols, implementation was accomplished in the second quarter of 2008. Quantitative and qualitative evaluation with defined indicators was conducted for 3 months after implementation of the project. The following indicators were monitored:

1. Direct observation of patients by nursing and medical staffs
2. Concurrent chart audit with defined indicators
   a. Number of seizures
   b. Vital signs
   c. Number of times PRN medications are used (based on CIWA [alcohol] scale)
   d. Pain Assessment Scale
   e. Number of times detoxification protocols have to be readjusted
3. Qualitative focus group of nursing staff with open-ended interview questions

Outcome evaluation began with the implementation of the treatment protocols for a 3-month period. Qualitative outcome research in the form of a focus group of nurses was conducted in June 2008. All participants signed informed consent to be interviewed. Open-ended interview questions were posed. Responses were audiotaped and transcribed verbatim. Audiotapes were destroyed following transcription. A thematic analysis of the data was conducted. Study results were reported in July 2008.

The following section lists the sample detoxification treatment protocols. Protocols would be selected based on patient's symptoms, history of substance abuse including the length of time substances were used, amount of substance used, and usage patterns, i.e., daily versus twice weekly, etc.

SAMPLE ADULT ALCOHOL DETOXIFICATION PROTOCOL # 1

Standing Orders

Patient Name: ______________________________ ID#: ________________

1. Admit to:
2. Regular diet
3. Vital signs per policy
4. Administer 0.1 cm^3 intradermally to left forearm Tuberculin Purified Protein Derivative; repeat in 2 weeks when applicable.
5. Multivitamins 1 tablet orally daily for length of stay
6. Thiamine 100 mg orally twice daily for 5 days, then
7. Thiamine 100 mg orally once daily thereafter for length of stay
8. Librium 75 mg orally as initial dose, then
9. Librium 50 mg orally every 6 hours for 24 hours, then
10. Librium 35 mg orally every 6 hours for 24 hours, then
11. Librium 25 mg orally every 6 hours for 24 hours, then
12. Librium 10 mg orally every 6 hours for 24 hours, then discontinue
13. Librium 25 mg orally every 4 hours as needed based on signs and symptoms of withdrawal for 5 days
14. Hyoscyamine (Levsin) 0.125 mg sublingually every 6 hours as needed for abdominal cramps for 5 days
15. Hydroxyzine (Vistaril) 50 mg orally every 4 hours as needed for anxiety or agitation for length of stay
16. Forty-eight hours after discontinuation of the detoxification protocol Campral 333 mg (2 tablets) will be initiated orally 3 times per day
17. Trazodone 50 mg orally at bedtime as needed for insomnia for length of stay
18. May repeat trazodone 50 mg orally 1 additional dose 2 hours after the first dose if the first dose is not effective as needed for insomnia for length of stay
19. Forty-eight hours after discontinuation of the detoxification protocol give naltrexone 25 mg orally at bedtime × 3 days, then increase naltrexone to 50 mg once orally at bedtime thereafter
20. Vivitrol 380 mg intramuscular to the gluteal region once monthly if patient fails naltrexone oral challenge or if patient's liver enzymes are elevated. Notify medical staff to discuss Vivitrol therapy with the patient before initiation and also for written prescription.
21. Milk of Magnesia 30 cm^3 orally twice daily as needed for constipation for length of stay
22. Magnesium hydroxide/aluminum hydroxide (Maalox) 30 cm^3 orally twice daily as needed for indigestion for length of stay

(Continued)

23. Bismuth subsalicylate (Kaopectate) 30 cm^3 orally twice daily as needed for diarrhea for length of stay
24. Acetaminophen (Tylenol) 2 tablets orally 3 times daily as needed for headache and/or temperature above 101°F for length of stay
25. Ibuprofen (Motrin) 600 mg orally every 6 hours as needed for muscle aches and pain for length of stay
26. Guaifenesin (Robitussin) 10 mL orally every 4 hours as needed for cough for length of stay
27. Benzocaine/menthol lozenges (Cepacol) throat lozenges 1 orally every 4 hours as needed for sore throat for length of stay
28. Random urine drug screen (as determined by nursing)
29. Complete the CIWA (for alcohol) if considering administration of PRN detoxification medication.

Note: This protocol may be adjusted at any time by the Medical Staff.

Routine Labs:	____ CBC	____ Urinalysis
	____ SMAC	____ Urine Drug Screen
	____ Urine Pregnancy Test	____ Serum Pregnancy Test

Physician/APN Signature: ________________ Date: _________
Time: ________

SAMPLE ADULT ALCOHOL DETOXIFICATION PROTOCOL # 2

Standing Orders

Patient Name: ________________________ ID#: ___________________

1. Admit to:
2. Regular diet
3. Vital signs per policy
4. Administer 0.1 cm^3 intradermally to left forearm Tuberculin Purified Protein Derivative; repeat in 2 weeks when applicable.
5. Multivitamins 1 tablet orally daily for length of stay
6. Thiamine 100 mg orally twice daily for 5 days, then
7. Thiamine 100 mg orally once daily thereafter for length of stay
8. Librium 75 mg orally as initial dose, then
9. Librium 75 mg orally every 6 hours for 24 hours, then
10. Librium 50 mg orally every 6 hours for 24 hours, then
11. Librium 35 mg orally every 6 hours for 24 hours, then
12. Librium 25 mg orally every 6 hours for 24 hours, then

13. Librium 10 mg orally every 6 hours for 24 hours, then discontinue
14. Librium 25 mg orally every 4 hours as needed based on signs and symptoms of withdrawal for 5 days, then discontinue
15. Levsin 0.125 mg sublingually every 6 hours as needed for abdominal pain for 5 days
16. Vistaril 50 mg orally every 4 hours as needed for anxiety or agitation for length of stay
17. Forty-eight hours after discontinuation of the detoxification protocol Campral 333 mg (2 tablets) will be initiated orally 3 times per day
18. Forty-eight hours after discontinuation of the detoxification protocol give naltrexone 25 mg orally at bedtime × 3 days, then increase naltrexone to 50 mg once orally at bedtime thereafter
19. Vivitrol 380 mg intramuscular to the gluteal region once monthly if the patient fails naltrexone oral challenge or if the patient's liver enzymes are elevated

    Notify medical staff to discuss Vivitrol therapy with the patient before initiation and also for written prescription.
20. Trazodone 50 mg orally at bedtime as needed for insomnia for length of stay
21. May repeat trazodone 50 mg orally 1 additional dose 2 hours after the first dose if the first dose is not effective as needed for insomnia for length of stay
22. Milk of Magnesia 30 cm^3 orally twice daily as needed for constipation for length of stay
23. Maalox 30 cm^3 orally twice daily as needed for indigestion for length of stay
24. Kaopectate 30 cm^3 orally twice daily as needed for diarrhea for length of stay
25. Tylenol 2 tablets orally 3 times a day as needed for headache or temperature above 101°F for length of stay
26. Motrin 600 mg orally every 6 hours as needed for muscle aches or pain for length of stay
27. Robitussin 10 mL orally every 4 hours as needed for cough for length of stay
28. Cepacol throat lozenges 1 orally every 4 hours as needed for sore throat for length of stay
29. Random urine drug screen (as determined by nursing)
30. Complete the CIWA (for alcohol) if considering administration of PRN detoxification medication

Note: This protocol may be adjusted at any time by the Medical Staff.

Routine Labs:	____ CBC	____ Urinalysis
	____ SMAC	____ Urine Drug Screen
	____ Urine Pregnancy Test	____ Serum Pregnancy Test

Physician/APN Signature: ________________ Date: __________
Time: _________

(Continued)

SAMPLE ADULT ALCOHOL DETOXIFICATION PROTOCOL # 3

Standing Orders

Patient Name: ______________________________ ID#: ____________________

1. Admit to:
2. Regular diet
3. Vital signs per policy
4. Administer 0.1 cm^3 intradermally to left forearm Tuberculin Purified Protein Derivative; repeat in 2 weeks when applicable.
5. Multivitamins 1 tablet orally daily for length of stay
6. Thiamine 100 mg orally twice daily for 5 days, then
7. Thiamine 100 mg orally once daily thereafter for length of stay
8. Librium 75 mg orally as initial dose, then
9. Librium 75 mg orally every 6 hours for 24 hours, then
10. Librium 50 mg orally every 6 hours for 24 hours, then
11. Librium 35 mg orally every 6 hours for 24 hours, then
12. Librium 25 mg orally every 6 hours for 24 hours, then
13. Librium 10 mg orally every 6 hours for 24 hours, then discontinue
14. Librium 25 mg orally every 4 hours as needed based on signs and symptoms of withdrawal for 5 days, then discontinue
15. Levsin 0.125 mg sublingually every 6 hours as needed for abdominal cramps for 5 days
16. Vistaril 50 mg orally every 4 hours as needed for anxiety or agitation for length of stay
17. Forty-eight hours after discontinuation of the detoxification protocol Campral 333 mg (2 tablets) will be initiated orally 3 times per day
18. Forty-eight hours after discontinuation of the detoxification protocol give naltrexone 25 mg orally at bedtime × 3 days, then increase naltrexone to 50 mg once orally at bedtime thereafter
19. Vivitrol 380 mg intramuscular to the gluteal region once monthly if patient fails naltrexone oral challenge or if patient's liver enzymes are elevated

    Notify medical staff to discuss Vivitrol therapy with the patient before initiation and also for written prescription.
20. Trazodone 50 mg orally at bedtime as needed for insomnia for length of stay
21. May repeat trazodone 50 mg orally 1 additional dose 2 hours after the first dose if the first dose is not effective as needed for insomnia for length of stay
22. Clonidine 0.2 mg orally now, then
23. Clonidine 0.1 mg orally every 6 hours for 24 hours, then

24. Clonidine 0.1 mg orally every 8 hours for 24 hours, then
25. Clonidine 0.1 mg orally every 12 hours for 24 hours, then discontinue
26. Hold clonidine if systolic blood pressure is less than 100 mm Hg and/or heart rate is less than 50 bpm
27. Carbamazepine (Tegretol) 200 mg orally twice daily for length of stay
28. Serum Tegretol level in 5 days
29. Milk of Magnesia 30 cm^3 orally twice daily as needed for constipation for length of stay
30. Kaopectate 30 cm^3 orally twice daily as needed for diarrhea for length of stay
31. Tylenol 2 tablets orally 3 times a day as needed for headache or temperature above 101°F for length of stay
32. Motrin 600 mg orally every 6 hours as needed for muscle aches or pain for length of stay
33. Robitussin 10 mL orally every 4 hours as needed for cough for length of stay
34. Cepacol throat lozenges 1 orally every 4 hours as needed for sore throat for length of stay
35. Random urine drug screen (as determined by nursing)
36. Complete the CIWA (for alcohol) if considering administration of PRN detoxification medication

Note: This protocol may be adjusted at any time by the Medical Staff.

Routine Labs: ____ CBC ____ Urinalysis

____ SMAC ____ Urine Drug Screen

____ Urine Pregnancy Test ____ Serum Pregnancy Test

Physician/APN Signature: ________________ Date: __________

Time: _________

SAMPLE ADULT OPIATE DETOXIFICATION PROTOCOL # 1

Standing Orders

Patient Name: ____________________________ ID#: ____________________

1. Admit to:
2. Regular diet
3. Vital signs per policy
4. Administer 0.1 cm^3 intradermally to left forearm Tuberculin Purified Protein Derivative; repeat in 2 weeks when applicable

(Continued)

5. Multivitamins 1 tablet orally daily for length of stay
6. Thiamine 100 mg orally once daily for length of stay
7. Phenobarbital 120 mg orally for 1 dose as needed and may repeat dose once as needed within a 24-hour period
8. Phenobarbital 75 mg orally every 6 hours for 24 hours, then
9. Phenobarbital 60 mg orally every 6 hours for 24 hours, then
10. Phenobarbital 45 mg orally every 6 hours for 24 hours, then
11. Phenobarbital 30 mg orally every 6 hours for 24 hours, then
12. Phenobarbital 15 mg orally every 6 hours for 24 hours, then discontinue
13. Clonidine 0.1 mg orally every 6 hours for 48 hours, then
14. Clonidine 0.1 mg orally every 8 hours for 24 hours, then
15. Clonidine 0.1 mg orally every 12 hours for 24 hours, then discontinue
16. Hold clonidine if systolic blood pressure is less than 100 mm Hg or heart rate is less than 60 bpm
17. Levsin 0.125 mg sublingually every 6 hours as needed for abdominal cramps for 5 days
18. Vistaril 50 mg orally every 4 hours as needed for anxiety or agitation for length of stay
19. Trazodone 50 mg orally at bedtime as needed for insomnia for length of stay
20. May repeat trazodone 50 mg orally one additional dose 2 hours after the first dose if the first dose is not effective as needed for insomnia for length of stay
21. Methocarbamol (Robaxin) 1500 mg orally 3 times a day for 5 days
22. Cyclobenzaprine (Flexeril) 10 mg orally at bedtime for 5 days
23. Milk of Magnesia 30 cm^3 orally twice daily as needed for constipation for length of stay
24. Maalox 30 cm^3 orally twice daily as needed for indigestion for length of stay
25. Kaopectate 30 cm^3 orally twice daily as needed for diarrhea for length of stay
26. Tylenol 2 tablets orally 3 times a day as needed for headache or temperature above 101°F for length of stay
27. Motrin 600 mg orally every 6 hours as needed for muscle aches or pain for length of stay
28. Robitussin 10 mL orally every 4 hours as needed for cough for length of stay
29. Cepacol throat lozenges 1 orally every 4 hours as needed for sore throat for length of stay
30. Random urine drug screen (as determined by nursing)
31. Complete the Clinical Opiate Withdrawal Scale (COWS) (for opiates) if considering administration of PRN detoxification medication

32. Naltrexone 25 mg orally once daily at bedtime for 3 days, then increase naltrexone to 50 mg orally once daily thereafter for length of stay.
33. Do not administer initial dose of naltrexone until patient has been off all opioids for a 10-day period

Note: This protocol may be adjusted at any time by the Medical Staff.

Routine Labs: ___ CBC ___ Urinalysis
___ SMAC ___ Urine Drug Screen
___ Urine Pregnancy test ___ Serum Pregnancy test

Physician/APN Signature: ________________ Date: _________
Time: _______

SAMPLE ADULT OPIATE DETOXIFICATION PROTOCOL # 2

Standing Orders

Patient Name: ____________________________ ID#: ____________________

1. Admit to:
2. Regular diet
3. Vital signs per policy
4. Administer 0.1 cm^3 intradermally to left forearm Tuberculin Purified Protein Derivative; repeat in 2 weeks when applicable.
5. Multivitamins 1 tablet orally daily for length of stay
6. Thiamine 100 mg orally once daily for length of stay
7. Phenobarbital 120 mg orally for 1 dose as needed and may repeat dose once as needed within a 24-hour period
8. Phenobarbital 60 mg orally every 6 hours for 24 hours, then
9. Phenobarbital 45 mg orally every 6 hours for 24 hours, then
10. Phenobarbital 30 mg orally every 6 hours for 24 hours, then
11. Phenobarbital 15 mg orally every 6 hours for 24 hours, then discontinue
12. Phenobarbital 30 mg orally every 6 hours as needed based on the signs and symptoms of withdrawal for 5 days
13. Clonidine 0.1 mg orally every 6 hours for 48 hours, then
14. Clonidine 0.1 mg orally every 8 hours for 24 hours, then
15. Clonidine 0.1 mg orally every 12 hours for 24 hours, then discontinue
16. Hold clonidine if systolic blood pressure is less than 100 mm Hg or heart rate is less than 60 bpm
17. Levsin 0.125 mg sublingually every 6 hours as needed for abdominal cramps for 5 days

(Continued)

18. Vistaril 50 mg orally every 4 hours as needed for anxiety or agitation for length of stay
19. Robaxin 1500 mg orally 3 times a day for 5 days
20. Flexeril 10 mg orally at bedtime for 5 days
21. Trazodone 50 mg orally at bedtime as needed for insomnia for length of stay
22. May repeat trazodone 50 mg orally 1 additional dose 2 hours after the first dose if the first dose is not effective as needed for insomnia for length of stay
23. Milk of Magnesia 30 cm^3 orally twice daily as needed for constipation for length of stay
24. Maalox 30 cm^3 orally twice daily as needed for indigestion for length of stay
25. Kaopectate 30 cm^3 orally twice daily as needed for diarrhea for length of stay
26. Tylenol 2 tablets orally 3 times a day as needed for headache or temperature above 101°F for length of stay
27. Motrin 600 mg orally every 6 hours as needed for muscle aches or pain for length of stay
28. Robitussin 10 mL orally every 4 hours as needed for cough for length of stay
29. Cepacol throat lozenges 1 orally every 4 hours as needed for sore throat for length of stay
30. Random urine drug screen (as determined by nursing)
31. Complete the COWS (for opiates) if considering administration of PRN detoxification medication
32. Naltrexone 25 mg orally once daily at bedtime for 3 days, then increase naltrexone to 50 mg orally once daily thereafter for length of stay.
33. Do not administer initial dose of naltrexone until patient has been off all opioids for a 10-day period.

Note: This protocol may be adjusted at any time by the Medical Staff.

Routine Labs:	___ CBC	___ Urinalysis
	___ SMAC	___ Urine Drug Screen
	___ Urine Pregnancy test	___ Serum Pregnancy test

Physician/APN Signature: ________________ Date: _________
Time: _________

SAMPLE ADULT OPIATE DETOXIFICATION PROTOCOL # 3

Standing Orders

Patient Name: ____________________________ ID#. __________________

1. Admit to:
2. Regular diet
3. Vital signs per policy

4. Administer 0.1 cm^3 intradermally to left forearm Tuberculin Purified Protein Derivative; repeat in 2 weeks when applicable.
5. Multivitamins 1 tablet orally daily for length of stay
6. Thiamine 100 mg orally once daily for length of stay
7. Methadone 20 mg orally today
8. Reduce methadone daily by 5 mg until dose is 0 mg. Begin order 12 hours after initial dose of methadone.
9. Clonidine 0.1 mg orally every 6 hours for 24 hours, then reduce to
10. Clonidine 0.1 mg orally every 8 hours for 24 hours, then reduce to
11. Clonidine 0.1 mg orally every 12 hours for 24 hours, then discontinue
12. Hold clonidine if systolic blood pressure is less than 100 mm Hg or heart rate is less than 60 bpm
13. Librium 25 mg orally every 6 hours for 24 hours, then reduce to
14. Librium 25 mg orally every 8 hours for 24 hours, then reduce to
15. Librium 10 mg orally every 8 hours for 24 hours, then discontinue
16. Librium 25 mg orally every 6 hours as needed based on signs and symptoms of withdrawal for 5 days
17. Levsin 0.125 mg sublingually every 6 hours as needed for abdominal cramps for 5 days
18. Vistaril 50 mg orally every 4 hours as needed for anxiety or agitation for length of stay
19. Robaxin 1500 mg orally 3 times a day for 5 days
20. Flexeril 10 mg orally at bedtime for 5 days
21. Trazodone 50 mg orally at bedtime as needed for insomnia for length of stay
22. May repeat trazodone 50 mg orally 1 additional dose 2 hours after the first dose if the first dose is not effective as needed for insomnia for length of stay
23. Milk of Magnesia 30 cm^3 orally twice daily as needed for constipation for length of stay
24. Maalox 30 cm^3 orally twice daily as needed for indigestion for length of stay
25. Kaopectate 30 cm^3 orally twice daily as needed for diarrhea for length of stay
26. Tylenol 2 tablets orally 3 times a day as needed for headache or temperature above 101°F for length of stay
27. Motrin 600 mg orally every 6 hours as needed for muscle aches or pain for length of stay
28. Robitussin 10 mL orally every 4 hours as needed for cough for length of stay
29. Cepacol throat lozenges 1 orally every 4 hours as needed for sore throat for length of stay
30. Random urine drug screen (as determined by nursing)

(Continued)

31. Complete the COWS (for opiates) if considering administration of PRN detoxification medication
32. Naltrexone 25 mg orally once daily at bedtime for 3 days, then increase naltrexone to 50 mg orally once daily thereafter for length of stay.
33. Do not administer initial dose of naltrexone until patient has been off methadone and all opioids for a 10-day period.

Note: This protocol may be adjusted at any time by the Medical Staff.

Routine Labs:	___ CBC	___ Urinalysis
	___ SMAC	___ Urine Drug Screen
	___ Urine Pregnancy test	___ Serum Pregnancy test

Physician/APN Signature: ________________ Date: ___________
Time: _________

SAMPLE ADULT OPIATE DETOXIFICATION PROTOCOL # 4

Standing Orders

Patient Name: ______________________________ ID#: __________________

1. Admit to:
2. Regular diet
3. Vital signs per policy
4. Administer 0.1 cm^3 intradermally to left forearm Tuberculin Purified Protein Derivative; repeat in 2 weeks when applicable.
5. Multivitamins 1 tablet orally daily for length of stay
6. Thiamine 100 mg orally once daily for length of stay
7. Methadone 25 mg orally today
8. Reduce methadone daily by 5 mg until dose is 0 mg. Begin order 12 hours after the initial dose of methadone.
9. Clonidine 0.1 mg orally every 6 hours for 24 hours, then reduce to
10. Clonidine 0.1 mg orally every 8 hours for 24 hours, then reduce to
11. Clonidine 0.1 mg orally every 12 hours for 24 hours, then discontinue
12. Hold clonidine if systolic blood pressure is less than 100 mm Hg or heart rate is less than 60 bpm
13. Librium 25 mg orally every 6 hours for 24 hours, then reduce to
14. Librium 25 mg orally every 8 hours for 24 hours, then reduce to

15. Librium 10 mg orally every 8 hours for 24 hours, then discontinue
16. Librium 25 mg orally every 6 hours as needed based on signs and symptoms of withdrawal for 5 days
17. Levsin 0.125 mg sublingually every 6 hours as needed for abdominal cramps for 5 days
18. Vistaril 50 mg orally every 4 hours as needed for anxiety or agitation for length of stay
19. Robaxin 1500 mg orally 3 times a day for 5 days
20. Flexeril 10 mg orally at bedtime for 5 days
21. Trazodone 50 mg orally at bedtime as needed for insomnia for length of stay
22. May repeat trazodone 50 mg orally 1 additional dose 2 hours after the first dose if the first dose is not effective as needed for insomnia for length of stay
23. Milk of Magnesia 30 cm^3 orally twice daily as needed for constipation for length of stay
24. Maalox 30 cm^3 orally twice daily as needed for indigestion for length of stay
25. Kaopectate 30 cm^3 orally twice daily as needed for diarrhea for length of stay
26. Tylenol 2 tablets orally 3 times a day as needed for headache or temperature above 101°F for length of stay
27. Motrin 600 mg orally every 6 hours as needed for muscle aches or pain for length of stay
28. Robitussin 10 mL orally every 4 hours as needed for cough for length of stay
29. Cepacol throat lozenges 1 orally every 4 hours as needed/for sore throat for length of stay
30. Random urine drug screen (as determined by nursing)
31. Complete the COWS (for opiates) if considering administration of PRN detoxification medication
32. Naltrexone 25 mg orally once daily at bedtime for 3 days, then increase naltrexone to 50 mg orally once daily thereafter for length of stay.
33. Do not administer initial dose of naltrexone until patient has been off methadone and all opioids for a 10-day period.

Note: This protocol may be adjusted at any time by the Medical Staff.

Routine Labs: ___ CBC ___ Urinalysis ___ Urine Drug Screen
___ SMAC ___ Urine Pregnancy test ___ Serum Pregnancy test

Physician/APN Signature: _______________ Date: _________
Time: ________

(Continued)

SAMPLE ADULT OPIATE DETOXIFICATION PROTOCOL # 5

Standing Orders

Patient Name: ______________________ ID#: ______________

1. Admit to:
2. Diet: ____________________
3. Vital signs per policy
4. Administer 0.1 cm^3 intradermally to left forearm Tuberculin Purified Protein Derivative; repeat in 2 weeks when applicable.
5. Buprenorphine titration per physician order after last use of opiates is greater than 24 hours and per criteria in COWS scale.
6. Multivitamins 1 tablet orally daily for length of stay
7. Vistaril 50 mg orally every 6 hours as needed for anxiety or agitation for length of stay
8. Robaxin 1500 mg orally 3 times a day for 5 days
9. Flexeril 10 mg orally at bedtime for 5 days
10. Trazodone 50 mg orally at bedtime as needed for insomnia for length of stay
11. May repeat trazodone 50 mg orally 1 additional dose 2 hours after the first dose if the first dose is not effective as needed for insomnia for length of stay
12. Milk of Magnesia 30 cm^3 orally twice daily as needed for constipation for length of stay
13. Maalox 30 cm^3 orally twice daily as needed for indigestion for length of stay
14. Kaopectate 30 cm^3 orally twice daily as needed for diarrhea for length of stay
15. Tylenol 2 tablets orally 3 times a day as needed for headache or temperature above 101°F for length of stay
16. Motrin 600 mg orally every 6 hours as needed for muscle aches or pain for length of stay
17. Robitussin 10 mL orally every 4 hours as needed for cough for length of stay
18. Cepacol throat lozenges 1 orally every 4 hours as needed for sore throat for length of stay
19. Random urine drug screen (as determined by nursing)
20. Complete the COWS (for opiates) if considering administration of PRN detoxification medication

Note: This protocol may be adjusted at any time by the Medical Staff.

Routine Labs:	___ CBC	___ Urinalysis
	___ SMAC	___ Urine Drug Screen
	___ Urine Pregnancy test	___ Serum Pregnancy test

Physician/APN Signature: ______________ Date: __________
Time: __________

SAMPLE ADULT BENZODIAZEPINE DETOXIFICATION PROTOCOL # 1

Standing Orders

Patient Name: ______________________________ ID#: ______________________

1. Admit to:
2. Regular diet
3. Vital signs per policy
4. Administer 0.1 cm^3 intradermally to left forearm Tuberculin Purified Protein Derivative; repeat in 2 weeks when applicable.
5. Multivitamins 1 tablet orally daily for length of stay
6. Thiamine 100 mg orally once daily for length of stay
7. Phenobarbital 120 mg orally for 1 dose as needed and may repeat dose once as needed within a 24-hour period
8. Phenobarbital 75 mg orally every 6 hours for 24 hours, then
9. Phenobarbital 60 mg orally every 6 hours for 24 hours, then
10. Phenobarbital 45 mg orally every 6 hours for 24 hours, then
11. Phenobarbital 30 mg orally every 6 hours for 24 hours, then
12. Phenobarbital 15 mg orally every 6 hours for 24 hours, then discontinue
13. Phenobarbital 30 mg orally every 6 hours as needed based on signs and symptoms
14. Clonidine 0.1 mg orally every 6 hours for 48 hours, then
15. Clonidine 0.1 mg orally every 8 hours for 24 hours, then
16. Clonidine 0.1 mg orally every 12 hours for 24 hours, then discontinue
17. Hold clonidine if systolic blood pressure is less 100 mm Hg and/or heart rate is less than 60 bpm
18. Levsin 0.125 mg sublingually every 6 hours as needed for abdominal cramps for 5 days
19. Vistaril 50 mg orally every 4 hours as needed for anxiety or agitation for length of stay
20. Tegretol 200 mg orally twice daily for length of stay
21. Serum Tegretol level in 5 days
22. Seizure precautions
23. Trazodone 50 mg orally at bedtime as needed for insomnia for length of stay
24. May repeat trazodone 50 mg orally 1 additional dose 2 hours after the first dose if the first dose is not effective as needed for insomnia for length of stay
25. Milk of Magnesia 30 cm^3 orally twice daily as needed for constipation for length of stay

(Continued)

26. Maalox 30 cm^3 orally twice daily as needed for indigestion for length of stay
27. Kaopectate 30 cm^3 orally twice daily as needed for diarrhea for length of stay
28. Tylenol 2 tablets orally 3 times a day as needed for headache or temperature above 101°F for length of stay
29. Motrin 600 mg orally every 6 hours as needed for muscle aches or pain for length of stay
30. Robitussin 10 mL orally every 4 hours as needed for cough for length of stay
31. Cepacol throat lozenges 1 orally every 4 hours as needed for sore throat for length of stay
32. Random urine drug screen (as determined by nursing)

Note: This protocol may be adjusted at any time by the Medical Staff.

Routine Labs:	___ CBC	___ Urinalysis
	___ SMAC	___ Urine Drug Screen
	___ Urine Pregnancy test	___ Serum Pregnancy test

Physician/APN Signature: _______________ Date: __________
Time: _________

QUESTIONS

1. "Pulse Rate" is:
   a. A dependent variable
   b. An independent variable
   c. Not a variable
   d. A categoric variable
2. The independent variable(s) in the research question, "Is heart rate increased by epinephrine?" is:
   a. Heart rate
   b. Epinephrine
   c. Drug
   d. Outcome
3. The dependent variable(s) in the research question, "What is the effect of noise levels on postoperative pain or blood pressure fluctuations in ICU patients?" is:
   a. Blood pressure
   b. Postoperative pain
   c. Noise levels
   d. Blood pressure and postoperative pain

4. The dependent variable in the hypothesis, "Baccalaureate degree-prepared nurses will practice more rehabilitative research measures on a client in an ICU than will associate degree-prepared nurses" is:
   a. Associate-degree prepared nurses
   b. Baccalaureate degree-prepared nurses
   c. Rehabilitative nursing measures
   d. Type of educational background of the nurse
5. The purpose of an operational definition in a quantitative study is to:
   a. Assign numeric values to variables
   b. Specify how a variable will be defined and measured
   c. State the expected relationship between the variables under investigation
   d. Designate the overall plan by which the data will be collected
6. The "P" in PICOT represents:
   a. Research producers
   b. Patient population of interest
   c. Sample
   d. Research assistants
7. What is one of the most important items to have to implement an EBP project?
   a. Self-reports
   b. Literature reviews
   c. Ample evidence
   d. Physical measures
8. The "C" in PICOT represents:
   a. Manipulated variable
   b. Outcome variable
   c. Comparative group
   d. Research variable
9. Which level of evidence best represents a rigorous controlled clinical trial?
   a. Level I
   b. Level II
   c. Level III
   d. Level IV
10. Qualitative research does **not** use which of the following?
   a. Inferential statistics
   b. Descriptive statistics
   c. Thematic analysis
   d. Audiotaping verbatim

ANSWERS: 1-a, 2-b, 3-d, 4-c, 5-b, 6-b, 7-c, 8-c, 9-a, 10-a

Match the Following

1. Descriptive statistics ____	a. Experimental design
2. Inferential statistics ____	b. Qualitative design
3. Outcome variable ____	c. Plan for research
4. True random sample ____	d. Most frequently occurring number

5. Numbers ____ e. Studies the culture of nursing
6. Words ____ f. Independent variable
7. Mode ____ g. Quantitative research
8. Research design ____ h. Infers/suggests a causal relationship
9. Ethnography ____ i. Dependent variable
10. Manipulated variable ____ j. Describes data

ANSWERS: 1-j, 2-h, 3-i, 4-a, 5-g, 6-b, 7-d, 8-c, 9-e, 10-f

True or False

1. The most frequently occurring number in a data set is the median. ____
2. The arithmetic average is the mode. ____
3. The median is the half way point. ____
4. An example of nominal data is the number on a football jersey. ____
5. Interval data has a consistent measurable distance. ____
6. Ratio data have an absolute zero point. ____
7. A pain scale is representative of ordinal data. ____
8. A quasi-experimental design lacks a true random sample. ____
9. Qualitative designs make extensive use of inferential statistics. ____
10. It is important to eliminate bias in a quantitative design. ____
11. Deductive reasoning starts with the specific and broadens. ____
12. Inductive reasoning starts with a broad definition and narrows. ____
13. Epistemology is the study of knowledge. ____
14. Practice change should be based on ritual. ____
15. Use of a true random sample allows for generalizability. ____

ANSWERS: 1-F, 2-F, 3-T, 4-T, 5-T, 6-T, 7-T, 8-T, 9-F, 10-T, 11-F, 12-F, 13-T, 14-F, 15-T

References

Brown, B. (1973). Use of alcohol by addict and non-addict populations. *American Journal of Psychology*, *130*, 599–601.

Caputo, F., Addolorato, G., Domenicali, M., Mosti, A., Viaggi, M., Trevisani, F., et al. (2002). Short-term methadone administration reduces alcohol consumption in non-alcoholic heroin addicts. *Alcohol and Alcoholism*, *37*(2), 164–168.

Carroll, K. M., Ball, S. A., Nich, C., O'Connor, P. G., Eagan, D. A., Frankforter, T. L., et al. (2001). Targeting behavioral therapies to enhance naltrexone treatment of opioid dependence. *Archives of General Psychiatry*, *58*, 755–761.

El-Bassel, N., Shilling, R. F., Turnbull, J. E., & Su, K. H. (1993). Correlates of alcohol use among methadone patients. *Alcoholism: Clinical and Experimental Research*, *17*, 681–686.

Fiellin, D. A., Rosenheck, R. A., & Kosten, T. R. (2001). Office-based treatment of opioid dependence: Reaching new patient populations. *American Journal of Psychiatry, 158*(8), 1200–1204.

Lejoyeux, M., Solomon, J., & Ades, J. (1998). Benzodiazepine treatment for alcohol dependent patients. *Alcohol and Alcoholism, 33*(6), 563–575.

Liebson, I., Bigelow, G., & Flamer, R. (1973). Alcoholism among methadone patients: A specific treatment method. *American Journal of Psychiatry, 130*, 483–485.

Melnyk, B., & Fineout-Overholt, E. (2014). *Evidence based practice in nursing and health care* (3rd ed.). Philadelphia, PA: Lippincott.

Nimmerrichter, A. A., Walter, H., Gutierrez-Lobos, K. E., & Lesch, O. M. (2002). Double-blind controlled trial of hydroxybutyrate and clomethiazole in the treatment of alcohol withdrawal. *Alcohol and Alcoholism, 37*(1), 67–73.

Ott, P. J., Tarter, R. E., & Ammerman, R. T. (Eds.). (1999). *Sourcebook on substance abuse: Etiology, epidemiology, assessment and treatment.* Boston, MA: Allyn and Bacon.

Phillips, S., Haycock, C., & Boyle, D. (2006). Development of an alcohol withdrawal protocol: CNS collaborative exemplar. *Clinical Nurse Specialist, 20*(4), 190–198.

Polit, D. F., & Beck, C. T. (2017). *Nursing research: Generating and assessing evidence for nursing practice.* Philadelphia, PA: Lippincott.

Streeton, C., & Whelan, G. (2001). Naltrexone, a relapse prevention maintenance treatment of alcohol dependence: A meta-analysis of randomized control trials. *Alcohol and Alcoholism, 36*(6), 544–552.

CHAPTER

4

Systems Thinking

William J. Lorman

This chapter will review:

SYSTEMS THEORY

CONCEPTS RELATED TO SYSTEMS THEORY

SYSTEMS SCIENCE

SYSTEMS THINKING

BASIC PRINCIPLES OF SYSTEMS THINKING

SYSTEMIC LEADERSHIP

SYSTEMS THEORY

Systems theory is the interdisciplinary study of systems. A system is an entity with interrelated and interdependent parts. It is defined by its boundaries and is more than the sum of its parts (called subsystems). Change in one part of the system affects other parts and the whole system, with predictable patterns of behavior. Positive growth and adaptation of a system depends on how well the system is adjusted with its environment, and systems often exist to accomplish a common purpose. The goal of systems science is to systematically discover a system's dynamics, constraints, and conditions and elucidate principles such as purpose, measure, methods, and tools that can be discerned and applied to systems at every level of nesting, and in every field for achieving optimized finality (Katok, Hasselblatt, & Katok, 1996). Some key concepts related to systems theory include the following:

- System—an organized entity made up of interrelated and interdependent parts
- Boundaries—barriers that define a system and distinguish it from other systems in the environment

- Homeostasis—the tendency of a system to resist change and maintain status quo
- Adaptation—the tendency of a system to make the changes needed to protect itself and grow to accomplish its goal
- Reciprocal transactions—circular interactions that systems engage in such that they influence one another
- Feedback loop—the process by which systems self-correct based on reactions from other systems in the environment
- Microsystem—the system closest to the client
- Mesosystem—relationships among the systems in an environment
- Exosystem—a relationship between 2 systems that has an indirect effect on a third system
- Macrosystem—a larger system that influences clients, such as policies, administration of entitlement programs, and culture
- Chronosystem—a system composed of significant life events that can affect adaptation

SYSTEMS SCIENCE

Systems thrive when all of their functions and dynamics intersect in the continual interactions of relationship and transformation. Systems science is based on the belief that the universe operates as a set of interacting forces and interdependent relationships. Everything in the universe is in some way acting on or interacting with something else. In this era of intersections, interactions, interdependencies, and horizontal linkages, the entire infrastructure of work has been altered as has our current understanding of the mechanics necessary to facilitate effective work. This has caused a movement from institutions to systems (Porter-O-Grady & Malloch, 2015).

SYSTEMS THINKING

Systems thinking, introduced by Senge (1990), uses habits, tools, and concepts to develop an understanding of the interdependent structures of dynamic systems. When individuals have a better understanding of systems, they are better able to identify the leverage points that lead to desired outcomes. Systems thinking can be envisioned as a vantage point from which a network of relationships is seen as a whole rather than focusing only on the detail of any particular piece, and as such, events are seen in the larger context of a pattern that is unfolding over time. It is a perspective of seeing and understanding systems as a whole rather than as collections of parts—a web of interconnections that creates emerging patterns.

Senge (1990) identifies 5 disciplines that must be embraced to become a learning organization:

1. Personal mastery is defined as the discipline of continually clarifying and deepening our personal vision, focusing our energies, developing patience, and seeing reality objectively.
2. Mental models are deeply ingrained assumptions, generalizations, or pictures of images that influence how we understand the world and how we take action.
3. Building shared vision is the practice of creating a shared picture of the future that fosters genuine commitment and engagement rather than compliance.
4. Team learning starts with dialogue and the capacity of the team to suspend assumptions and think together.
5. Systems thinking integrates all the previous disciplines.

Systems thinking strategies fall into 3 general categories: visual, listening and speaking, and kinesthetic. All 3 categories, especially when applied together, help people practice the habits of a systems thinker, building capacity to think systemically over time. The visual tools of systems thinking include the use of graphs, diagrams, and other visual content. Visual tools help the individual collect, analyze, synthesize, and communicate his or her thoughts about systems. Listening and speaking strategies depend on the development of a common vocabulary and the use of different communication techniques to increase understanding of how systems work by increasing the ability to see a bigger picture through multiple perspectives. Finally, kinesthetic strategies engage the body along with the mind to study how and why a system functions as it does.

The approach of systems thinking is fundamentally different from that of traditional forms of analysis. Traditional analysis focuses on separating the individual pieces of what is being studied and then studying each part. Systems thinking, in contrast, focuses on how the thing being studied interacts with the other constituents of the system. Stated another way, instead of isolating smaller and smaller parts of the system being studied, systems thinking works by expanding its view to take into account larger and larger numbers of interactions as an issue is being studied. This often results in strikingly different conclusions than those generated by traditional forms of analysis. This is especially true when what is being studied is dynamically complex or has a great deal of feedback from other sources, be they internal or external. The character of systems thinking makes it extremely effective on the most difficult types of problems to solve, for example, those involving complex issues, those that have a great deal of dependence on past actions or on the actions of others, and those stemming from ineffective coordination among those involved. Examples of areas in which systems thinking has proved its value include the following:

- Complex problems that involve helping many individuals see the "big picture" and not just their part of it
- Recurring problems or those that have been made worse by past attempts to fix them
- Issues where an action affects or is affected by the environment surrounding the issue, either the natural environment or the competitive environment
- Problems whose solutions are not obvious

BASIC PRINCIPLES OF SYSTEMS THINKING

In his discussion of Leadership and Systems, Tate (2009) states that systems thinking is a management discipline that requires an understanding of a system by examining the linkages and interactions between the components that comprise the entirety of the system that is being defined. The whole system is a systems thinking view of the complete organization in relation to its environment. It provides a means of understanding, analyzing, and talking about the design and construction of the organization as an integrated, complex composition of many interconnected systems (human and nonhuman) that need to work together for the whole to function successfully. Systems can have clear external boundaries—called closed systems—or have links with their environment—called open systems. An open systems perspective is the more common and realistic.

An organization can suffer systemic failure. This occurs when there is a failure between and within the system elements that need to work together for overall success. Some examples of factors in systemic failure are confused goals, weak system-wide understanding, flawed design, individual incentives that encourage loyalty to subordinate rather than superordinate goals, inadequate feedback, poor cooperation, and lack of accountability. System success requires a performance management system that is propelled above the level of individual systems and their functional leadership. Features may include group or team-level goal setting, development, incentives, communication, reviews, rewards, and accountability. The aim is to focus on what binds individuals together and what binds systems together rather than functional silo performance. System failure may coexist alongside functional success. The leadership of silos may individually be successful but not be sufficiently integrated into the whole system owing to a shortcoming of systems design, management, or understanding.

The system can succeed only through collaboration of managers in and across a number of functional systems. The system will fail only if leadership at the level of the whole system fails, and where several senior managers are involved. Understanding and anticipating how the whole system is intended to work, how it actually works, and how it may buckle under pressure can elude and defeat most executives. The leadership challenge is emphasized by the realization that for every legitimate, official, or consciously designed system, there is a shadow system where all the nonrational issues reside, such as politics, trust, hopes, ambitions, greed, favors, and power struggles.

SYSTEMIC LEADERSHIP

Systemic leadership captures 2 important ideas: First, it is the leadership of an organization conceived of, understood, and managed by senior managers as a system, and second, it is the application of aspects of systems thinking to the subject of leadership. The systemic approach can be thought of as follows:

1. Developing the organization's systemic leadership capability
2. Expanding the organization's leadership capacity
3. Linking leadership development with business aims and objectives
4. Aligning leadership with where the organization is going
5. Uniting and building corporate leadership cohesion and spirit
6. Addressing conflicting perceptions of leadership in the organization
7. Merging leaders' individual and collective accountability
8. Solving precarious leadership problems (e.g., shortage of leaders)
9. Stopping the waste of leadership talent

We can all become better systems thinkers by being inquisitive, becoming knowledgeable beyond our own discipline, and asking questions about the relationships among events (Sherman, 2014). The following is an example of where systems thinking was used:

> *A healthcare organization was looking to change the way nursing staff entered medical histories so they could be integrated directly with patients' problem lists so that medical histories would no longer be stand-alone data elements. Rather, nursing would enter patient histories as patients stated their problems. After the system was activated, it was discovered that the change impacted physician billing because the medical history collected by nursing was used by billers to generate additional charges. There was a direct impact on revenue capture that was not considered prior to the change.*
>
> (Adapted from Roussel, L., Thomas, P. L., & Harris, J.L. [2016]. *Management and leadership for nurse administrators* [7th ed.]. Burlington, MA: Jones & Bartlett Learning. p. 291.)

CONCLUSION

Many important problems that plague us today are complex, involve multiple players, and are at least partly the result of past actions that were taken to alleviate them. Dealing with such problems is notoriously difficult, and the results of conventional solutions are often poor enough to create discouragement about the prospects of ever effectively addressing them. One of the key benefits of systems thinking is its ability to deal effectively with just these types of problems and to raise our thinking to the level at which we create the results we want as individuals and organizations even in those difficult situations marked by complexity, great numbers of interactions, and the absence or ineffectiveness of immediately apparent solutions (Senge, 1990).

QUESTIONS

1. Individual parts of a system are called a:
   a. Microsystem
   b. Subsystem
   c. Ubersystem
   d. Partial system
2. A relationship between 2 systems that has an indirect effect on a third system is called a(n):
   a. Microsystem
   b. Mesosystem
   c. Macrosystem
   d. Exosystem
3. The category of systems thinking strategies that uses graphs and diagrams is known as:
   a. Visual
   b. Listening and speaking
   c. Kinesthetic
   d. Neurolinguistics
4. An area where systems thinking has proved its value is:
   a. Complex problems that involve helping the individual see his or her part of the "big picture"
   b. Problems whose solutions are obvious
   c. Problems that have been made worse by past attempts to fix them
   d. Issues where actions affect the environment minimally
5. An example of a factor leading to systems failure is:
   a. Communication
   b. Accountability
   c. Individual incentives
   d. Reviews

ANSWERS: 1-b, 2-d, 3-a, 4-c, 5-c

References

Katok, A., Hasselblatt, B., & Katok, A. B. (1996). *Introduction to the modern theory of dynamical systems*. New York: Cambridge University Press.

Porter-O-Grady, T., & Malloch, K. (2015). *Quantum leadership: Building better partnerships for sustainable health* (4th ed.). Burlington, MA: Jones & Bartlett Learning.

Roussel, L., Thomas, P. L., & Harris, J. L. (2016). *Management and leadership for nurse administrators* (7th ed.; p. 291). Burlington, MA: Jones & Bartlett Learning.

Senge, P. (1990). *The fifth discipline*. New York: Doubleday.

Sherman, R. O. (2014). *Becoming a systems thinker*. Retrieved from http://www.emergingrnleader.com/systemsthinkinginnursing/.

Tate, W. (2009). *The search for leadership: An organizational perspective*. Charmouth Dorset: Triarchy Press.

CHAPTER

5

Strategic Management

William J. Lorman

This chapter will review:

FORMING A STRATEGIC VISION

SETTING OBJECTIVES

CRAFTING A STRATEGY TO ACHIEVE THE DESIRED OUTCOMES

IMPLEMENTING AND EXECUTING THE CHOSEN STRATEGY

EVALUATING PERFORMANCE, MONITORING NEW DEVELOPMENTS, AND INITIATING CORRECTIVE ADJUSTMENTS

EXTERNAL FACTORS THAT AFFECT STRATEGIC MANAGEMENT

INTERNAL FACTORS THAT AFFECT STRATEGIC MANAGEMENT

THE PROCESS OF STRATEGIC ANALYSIS

TESTS USED IN CONSIDERING BEST STRATEGIES

IMPLEMENTATION STRATEGIES

PLANNING IN A DYNAMIC ENVIRONMENT

LONG-RANGE PLANNING VERSUS STRATEGIC PLANNING

STRATEGIC PLANNING VERSUS STRATEGIC MANAGEMENT

STRATEGIC MANAGEMENT VERSUS HEALTH POLICY PLANNING

MANAGEMENT MODELS, APPROACHES, AND TECHNIQUES OVER THE YEARS

There are 5 tasks required for a strategic planning process. The first is **forming a strategic vision**, the earliest phase where a set of pertinent questions must be answered. For example,

- What is the vision for the organization?
- Where should the organization be headed?
- What should its future focus be?

- What kind of enterprise do you want to become?
- What do you want to achieve in 5 years?

The second task is **setting objectives**. The purpose of setting objectives is to convert managerial statements of strategic vision and business mission into specific performance targets that include the results and outcomes the organization wants to achieve. After objectives are set, there must be a means of measuring whether they are achieved or not to help track progress. Objectives can be specific to a particular perspective. Examples include the following:

- Financial objectives, such as improving cost efficiency and increasing revenue growth
- Customer objectives, such as expanding market share and enhancing brand image such as "Centers of Excellence"
- Internal process objectives, such as achieving operational excellence, driving demand through customer relation management, managing growth through innovation, and implementing good environmental policy
- Learning and growth objectives, such as developing strategic competencies, building learning culture, and expanding capabilities with technology

The third task is **crafting a strategy to achieve the desired outcomes**. This strategy represents management's answers to fundamental business questions such as the following:

- Whether to concentrate on a single entity or build a diversified group of entities
- Whether to cater to a broad range of customers or focus on a particular market niche
- How to respond to changing buyer preferences
- How to determine the geographic market
- How to react to newly emerging markets and competition
- How to grow the enterprise over the long term

The fourth task is **implementing and executing the chosen strategy**. Implementation refers to the managerial exercise of putting a freshly chosen strategy into place; execution deals with the managerial exercise of supervising the ongoing pursuit of strategy, making it work, and showing measurable progress in achieving the targeted results.

The fifth task is **evaluating performance, monitoring new developments, and initiating corrective adjustments**. Managers must stay on top of the organization's situation, deciding whether things are going well internally and monitoring outside developments closely. Marginal performance or too little progress, as well as important new external circumstances, requires corrective actions and adjustments.

There are many factors that shape the choice of strategy—both external and internal factors. It is the mix of considerations that determine an organization's strategic situation. Examples of external factors include the following:

- **Economic, societal, political, and government regulations.** What an organization can and cannot do is always constrained by what is legal, by what complies with government policies and regulatory requirements, by what is considered ethical, and by what is in accord with societal expectations and the standards of good social and community citizenship.
- **Competitive conditions and industry attractiveness.** An organization's competitive conditions and overall attractiveness are big strategy-determining factors, and strategies have to be tailored to the nature and mix of competitive factors in play, such as price, quality, and performance features.
- **Company opportunities and threats.** The organization's strategies need to be deliberately aimed at capturing its best growth opportunities, especially the ones that hold the most promise for building sustainable competitive advantage and enhancing profitability. Strategies should also provide a defense against external threats to the organization's well-being and future performance.

Examples of internal factors include the following:

- **Organizational strengths and weaknesses, competencies, and capabilities.** One of the most pivotal strategy-shaping internal considerations is whether an organization has or can acquire the resources, competencies, and capabilities needed to execute a strategy proficiently. The best path to competitive advantage is found where the organization has competitively valuable resources and competencies, where competitors cannot develop comparable capabilities except at high cost or over an extended period.
- **Personal ambitions and business philosophies of key executives.** Executives are typically influenced by their own vision of how to compete and how to position the organization and by what image and standing they want the organization to have.
- **Shared values and organizational culture.** The organization's policies, practices, traditions, philosophical beliefs, and ways of doing things combine to create a distinctive culture. The stronger an organization's culture, the more that culture is likely to shape the company's strategic actions, sometimes even dominating the choice of strategic moves.

The process of strategic analysis includes asking questions about the organization's industry and competitive conditions and also its own situation.

When considering the industry and competitive conditions, key questions include the following:

- What are the industry's dominant economic features?
- What is causing the industry's competitive structure and business environment to change?
- Which organizations are in the strongest/weakest positions?
- What strategic moves are competitors likely to make next?
- What are the key factors for competitive success?
- Is the industry attractive and what are the prospects for above-average profitability?

When considering the organization's own situation, key questions include the following:

- How well is the organization's present strategies working?
- What are the organization's strengths, weaknesses, opportunities, and threats?
- Are the organization's fees and/or contractual rates competitive?
- How strong is the organization's competitive position?
- What strategic issues does the organization face?

When considering best strategies, there are 3 tests. The first is the **goodness of fit test**. A good strategy has to be well matched to industry and competitive conditions, market opportunities and threats, and other aspects of the organization's external environment. At the same time, it has to be tailored to the organization's resource strengths and weaknesses, competencies, and competitive capabilities. The second test is the **competitive advantage test**. A good strategy leads to sustainable competitive advantage. The bigger the competitive edge that a strategy helps build, the more powerful and effective it is. The third test is the **performance test**. A good strategy boosts the organization's performance. There are 2 kinds of performance improvements that are the most telling of a strategy's caliber: gains in profitability and gains in the organization's competitive strength and long-term market position.

There are many considerations when implementing a strategic plan:

1. **How capable is the organization**? Is there a strong management team? Is there a mechanism for recruiting and retaining talented employees?
2. **Is there a strategy-supportive reward system**? Strategy-supportive motivational practices and reward systems are powerful tools for gaining employee buy-in and commitment. The key to creating a reward system that promotes good strategy execution is to make strategically relevant measures of performance the basis for designing incentives, evaluating individual and group efforts, and handing out rewards.

3. **Is there a strategy-supportive corporate culture?** Building a strategy-supportive culture is important to successful strategy execution because it produces a work climate and organizational solidarity that thrives on meeting performance targets.
4. **Is strategic leadership present**? Strategic leaders encourage people to be innovative to keep the organization responsive to changing conditions, alert to new opportunities, and anxious to pursue fresh initiatives. Strategic leaders also actively push corrective actions to improve strategy execution and overall strategic performance.
5. **Does the budget support the strategy**? Reworking the budget to make it more strategy-supportive is a crucial part of the implementation process because every organization needs to have the people, equipment, facilities, and other resources to carry out its part of the strategic plan.
6. **Have strategy-supportive policies and procedures been established?** Instituting new or revised policies and operating procedures aids the task of implementation by promoting consistency in how particular strategy-critical activities are performed throughout the organization's operating units and also by helping to create a strategy-supportive work climate and corporate culture.
7. **Is there a plan for continuous improvement**? Competent strategy execution entails visible, unyielding managerial commitment to best practices and continuous improvement. Benchmarking and the identification and adoption of best practices aim at improved efficiency, better services, and greater customer satisfaction.
8. **Is there an information system to support strategy execution**? Organizational strategies cannot be implemented well without a well-conceived state-of-the-art support system that not only facilitates better strategy execution but also strengthens organizational capabilities enough to provide a competitive edge.

PLANNING IN A DYNAMIC ENVIRONMENT

Health care leaders are often perplexed by certain questions in preparation for strategic planning. Some areas are as follows:

- How can organizations deal with important, complex, and sometimes conflicting issues and trends?
- Which ones are most important or most pressing? How difficult is it to prioritize?
- What new issues might emerge within health care's dynamic environment?

It is likely that there will be new opportunities and threats to health care organizations that have yet to be identified or fully assessed. In addition, it seems certain that there will be more change in the industry in the next 10 years than there has been in the past 10 years. Organizational change most definitely is a fundamental part of survival. In an environment of rapid, complex, and often discontinuous change, organizations must understand the nature and implications of external change, the ability to develop effective strategies that account for change, and the will as well as the ability to actively manage the momentum of the organization.

LONG-RANGE PLANNING VERSUS STRATEGIC PLANNING

The objective of long-range planning is to predict for some specified time in the future the size of demand for an organization's products and services and to determine where demand will occur. Long-range planning developed in the 1950s because operating budgets were difficult to prepare without some idea of future sales and the flow of funds. After World War II, economies were growing and the demand for many products and services was accelerating. Long-range forecasts of demand enabled managers to develop detailed marketing and distribution, production, human resources, and financial plans for growing organizations. Many organizations have used long-range planning to determine facilities expansion, hiring forecasts, capital needs, etc.

As businesses became somewhat more dynamic and volatile, long-range planning was replaced by strategic planning because the assumption underlying long-range planning is that the organization will continue to produce its present products and services, and so matching production capacity to demand became the critical issue. However, an added concern is that there is so much economic, social, political, technologic, and competitive change taking place that the organization must periodically evaluate whether it should even be offering its present products and services, whether it should start offering different products and services, or whether it should be operating and marketing in a fundamentally different way.

STRATEGIC PLANNING VERSUS STRATEGIC MANAGEMENT

During the 1960s and 1970s, there was major growth and strategic planning was the new rule. The process of strategic planning provided more systematic approaches to managing business units and extended the planning and budgeting horizon beyond the traditional 12-month operating period. In the 1980s the concept of strategic planning was broadened to strategic management. This evolutionary change acknowledged not only the importance of the dynamics of the environment and that organizations may have to totally reinvent themselves but also that continuously managing and evaluating the strategy were the foundation for success.

STRATEGIC MANAGEMENT VERSUS HEALTH POLICY PLANNING

Strategic management is organization specific and helps the organization respond to various state and federal policy and planning efforts. The intent of health policy is to provide the context for the development of the health care infrastructure as a whole.

MANAGEMENT MODELS, APPROACHES, AND TECHNIQUES OVER THE YEARS

Over the years, there have been multiple management approaches, as shown here, that attempted to change and improve the organization in areas such as to improve quality, to improve employee morale, to do more with less, to put meaning into work, and to focus efforts. The goals for all of the approaches were to manage and shape the organization to make it better. Many of these approaches are common and well known, others not so much. The reader can research any of these models to find out the positives and negatives of each:

The 1950s

- Theory X versus theory Y
- Management by objectives
- Quantitative management
- Diversification

The 1960s

- Managerial grid
- T-groups
- Matrix management
- Conglomeration
- Centralization versus decentralization

The 1970s

- Zero-based budgets
- Participative management

- Portfolio management
- Quantitative MBAs

The 1980s

- Theory Z
- One-minute managing
- Organizational culture
- Intrapreneuring
- Downsizing
- Management by wandering around
- Total quality management versus continuous quality improvement

The 1990s

- Customer focus
- Quality improvement
- Reengineering
- Benchmarking
- Resource-based view

The 2000s

- Six Sigma
- Balanced scorecard
- Transformational leadership
- Servant leadership
- Self-managed teams
- Dynamic capabilities
- Virtual organizations

CONCLUSIONS

Strategic management is a complex and difficult task. As we move forward in the 21st century, there will be a higher premium on effective strategic management and leadership than ever before, and no single approach may be adequate to understand the social and organizational processes that occur in the health care environment. Indeed, different leadership styles may be necessary depending on the organizational situation at hand. And experience has demonstrated that strategic management is not always a structured, well-thought-out exercise. Thought does not always precede action; perfect information about the environment and organization never exists; and rationality and logic are not always superior to intuition and luck. Organizations sometimes "do" before they "know." An astute leader realizes that, once introduced, strategies are subject to a variety of forces, both within and outside the organization. And sometimes we learn just by doing (Swayne, Duncan, & Ginter, 2006).

QUESTIONS

1. Which of the following would not be an objective in the strategic management process?
   a. To achieve operational excellence
   b. To expand market share
   c. To improve staff morale
   d. To implement an effective environmental policy
2. Reacting to newly emerging competition is an example of a(n):
   a. Strength
   b. Weakness
   c. Opportunity
   d. Threat
3. The task most often minimized or forgotten in the strategic management process is:
   a. Creating a strategic vision
   b. Considering effects on revenue generation
   c. Identifying technology issues
   d. Evaluating performance outcomes
4. Strategic analysis of the external and internal environments includes all of the following except:
   a. How strong is the organization's competitive position?
   b. How can the organization avoid competitors' actions?
   c. What are the industry's dominant economic features?
   d. What strategic issues does the organization face?
5. Which of the following tests is used when considering best strategies?
   a. The goodness of fit test
   b. The competitor avoidance test
   c. The capital gains test
   d. The depreciation test
6. An issue in the health care arena that is often ignored is:
   a. How difficult is it to prioritize?
   b. How are conflicting issues and trends handled?
   c. What issues may emerge in the future that cause concern?
   d. What issues are important to address strategically?
7. The notion that organizations must continuously manage and evaluate their strategies is an example of:
   a. Long-range planning
   b. Strategic planning
   c. Strategic management
   d. Health policy planning

ANSWERS: 1-c, 2-d, 3-d, 4-b, 5-a, 6-c, 7-c

References

Swayne, L. E., Duncan, W. J., & Ginter, P. M. (2006). *Strategic management of health care organizations* (5th ed.). Malden, MA: Blackwell Publishing.

CHAPTER

6

Human Resources

William J. Lorman

This chapter will review:

HUMAN RESOURCES IN THE HEALTH CARE INDUSTRY

HR PLANNING AND JOB ANALYSIS

STAFFING

TRAINING AND ORGANIZATIONAL DEVELOPMENT

PERFORMANCE MANAGEMENT AND COMPENSATION

EMPLOYEE RIGHTS

CHARACTERISTICS OF HIGH-PERFORMING ORGANIZATIONS

ENVIRONMENTAL TRENDS

THE JOINT COMMISSION AND HUMAN RESOURCES

EMPLOYMENT LAW

STATUS OF EMPLOYMENT

EMPLOYEE RELATIONS

PROFESSIONALISM: HAVING KNOWLEDGE AND SKILLS

HEALTH CARE PROFESSIONALS

CONSIDERATIONS FOR HR MANAGEMENT

UNIONS, UNIONIZATION, AND MANAGING THE RELATIONSHIPS

INTRODUCTION

Human resources (HR), along with financial resources and physical resources, are necessary elements required in the development, implementation, and maintenance of an organization and its goals. Organizations are composed of people, and these people represent one of the organization's most valuable assets. But the resource is seldom given any importance because the organization does not own people like its other capital and physical assets. Human resource management (HRM) is defined as a set of policies, practices, and programs designed to optimize both personal and organizational goals. One primary function is to assist managers in the recruitment, selection, and development of staff for the organization. This department is also important in the evaluation and compensation of employees along with attending to their labor relations, health and safety, and fairness concerns.

The evolution of the HRM movement began in the 1890s, and through the time of World War I, the managers were known as "Labor Managers," and after World War II, they were organized as a department whose main function was "to procure and develop" personnel. During the 1970s, the department was referred to as personnel management. During the 1980s and 1990s, the name was changed to human resource management, and in addition to procuring and developing employees, they were also tasked with motivating them. At present, the functions of the HR department are generally found at the vice president level of larger organizations and the staff are referred to as HR specialists. Additional tasks of this department at many organizations include legal compliance activities and, where present, union-management relations.

HUMAN RESOURCES IN THE HEALTH CARE INDUSTRY

Today, health care executives must understand the factors that influence the performance of the employees in their organizations to effectively manage them. These factors include not only the traditional HRM activities but also the environmental and other organizational aspects that affect HR activities. Strategic HRM is the process of formulating HR strategies and implementation tactics that are aligned and reinforcing the organization's business strategy. A significant trend that has recently developed is for HR managers to adopt a strategic perspective in their job and to recognize critical linkages between organizational strategy and HR strategy.

A number of HR practices are often found in organizations that are effective in managing their HR and enhance the health care organization's overall performance (Platonova & Hernandez, 2013). Some of the practices found to be especially effective for health care organizations include the following:

- **HR planning and job analysis.** The HR executive encourages employee involvement so that there can be strong buy-in with respect to managerial initiatives and practices. The HR executive also encourages teamwork to make employees more willing to collaborate through use of self-managed teams and decentralization to minimize management layers. Another important aspect of job analysis is to develop strategies to enhance employee work-life balance.

- **Staffing.** Be proactive in identifying and attracting talent. In selecting new employees, executives should use additional criteria beyond basic skills, such as attitudes, customer focus, and cultural fit.
- **Training and organizational development.** It is important to invest in training and organizational programs to enhance employee skills related to the organization's goals. Other initiatives include providing employees with future career opportunities by giving promotional priority to internal candidates and also include customer service in new employee onboarding and skills development.
- **Performance management and compensation.** Recognize employees by providing monetary and nonmonetary rewards and base individual and team compensation on goal-oriented results. Consider reducing status distinction and barriers, such as dress, office arrangement, parking, and wage differentials. Although usually a function of profitability, work toward offering high compensation contingent on organizational performance to reduce employee turnover and increase attraction to high-quality employees.
- **Employee rights.** Managers should communicate effectively with employees to keep them informed of major issues and initiatives, along with providing employment security for those who perform well, so that they are not downsized because of economic downturns or strategic errors by senior management. In addition, share financial and performance information to develop a high-trust organization.

No practices as identified earlier are "good" in and of themselves. Their impact always depends on how well the process fits the organization. Fit, or alignment, leads to better performance, whereas its lack creates inconsistencies. The overall performance of the organization is enhanced when HR practices are aligned with business strategy, are attuned to the external environment, enable the organization to capitalize on its distinctive capabilities, and reinforce one another. Wolf (2012) has identified 7 characteristics of high-performing health care organizations:

1. Visionary leadership
2. Consistent and effective communication
3. Selecting for fit and ongoing development of staff
4. Agile and open culture
5. Central focus on service

6. Constant recognition and broad community outreach
7. Solid physician/clinical relationships

It is the combination of these characteristics that helps health care organizations drive exceptional outcomes in patient experience, engagement, quality, and financial outcomes.

ENVIRONMENTAL TRENDS

There are multiple major environmental trends that affect health care organizations. The Society for Human Resource Management (2014) regularly surveys expert panels to review recent and future trends in HRM, such as the following:

- The continuing impact of the U.S. economy has created challenges that have affected budgets, hiring, and capital HR strategies.
- The need for skilled and educated workers is creating competition for those in highest demand, which influences all areas of HR.
- Ongoing developments in information and communication technologies, such as social media, have influenced recruiting and selection.
- Demographic changes have increased the percentage of aging employees and have increased diversity, affecting all aspects of HR practice.
- These demographic changes have caused employers to emphasize flexible and effective work-life strategies.
- Metrics and more in-depth data analysis are being required to demonstrate the return on investment of HR expenditures.
- The increase in uncertainty and market volatility have made uncertainty the new normal.
- The future of the Affordable Care Act, as well as the need to ensure compliance with a wide variety of federal and state laws, has created continuing challenges for HR managers.

The Equal Employment Opportunity Commission (2014) has identified that most of the growth in the capital HR function over the past few decades has been attributed to its crucial role in keeping organizations in compliance with laws and regulations promulgated by federal, state, and local governments as they relate to HR. The following are the 8 most significant HR environmental challenges as identified by Gomez-Mejia, Balkin, and Cardy (2012):

- Rapid change
- The rise of the Internet
- Workforce diversity
- Globalization
- Legislation

- Evolving work and family roles
- Skill shortages
- The rise of the service sector

In addition, the Society for Human Resource Management (2012) has projected that 3 major challenges in HR over the next 10 years will be retaining and rewarding the best employees, developing the next generation of corporate leaders, and creating an organizational culture that attracts the best employees.

THE JOINT COMMISSION AND HUMAN RESOURCES

The Joint Commission (TJC) requires health care organizations to continually screen for issues that can potentially arise as a result of inadequate staffing, with a focus on the link between adequate staffing and clinical outcomes. TJC requires a health care facility to select a minimum of 4 screening indicators, which must include 2 indicators for clinical or service issues and 2 for the HR function. Examples of HR screening indicators that define impact on the organization include areas such as amount of overtime, staff vacancy rates, turnover rates, nursing hours per patient-day, injuries on the job, use of per diem staff, and amount of sick time. The organization is expected to determine the causes of these indicators when the data vary from what is expected. If the problems are beyond the threshold, the organization undertakes steps leading to appropriate actions that will likely remedy the problems. Some strategies that might address identified staffing issues include recruitment efforts, continuing education and training, provision of additional support staff, and reorganization of workflow.

EMPLOYMENT LAW

Employment law affects and regulates HRM in many ways. For instance, Title VII of the 1964 Civil Rights Act prohibits discrimination in any "terms, conditions, or privileges of employment," and no court, in more than 50 years of litigation, has found an aspect of employment that is not covered by this prohibition. There are also many other regulations that prohibit discrimination. The Americans with Disabilities Action (ADA) and the Amendments Act (ADAAA) covers employees with disabilities and persons regarded as disabled; and for persons aged 40 years and older, there is the Aged Discrimination in Employment Act. Other HR activities such as hiring, promotions, transfers, opportunities for training, leave, payment of employees, discipline, termination, allegations of sexual harassment, and retaliation are all regulated by federal and state statutes, such as the Fair Labor Standards Act (FLSA), the Family and Medical Leave

Act (FMLA), the Genetic Information Nondiscrimination Act, and the Equal Employment Opportunity Commission (EEOC). Many states have enforced their own statutes, which are more restrictive than those of the Federal government, and leaders must not only be aware of and understand the Federal guidelines but also know what their state's statutes promulgate.

The broad language of Title VII (42 USC §2000e-2(a)(1)) covers any act or failure to act in every possible aspect of employment. The broad terminology allows interpretation even when faced with future technology so that, for example, employment discrimination in social media is still prohibited. Another provision of Title VII (§2000e(j)) requires the employer to "reasonably accommodate to an employee's or prospective employee's religious observance or practice." This section introduced the concept of reasonable accommodation, which is also promulgated in the ADA and the later ADAAA to cover other nonreligious areas of accommodation.

Beginning in the 1970s, the U.S. Supreme Court's role in the interpretation of the statutes has a long history of applying very broad criteria. For instance, in the landmark case of Griggs v. Duke Power Co. (401 US 424 (1971)), the Court established the concept of disparate impact. In this case, a power company had implemented promotional qualifications that included a requirement of a high school diploma, which ended up barring many African American employees. The Court found that, although this requirement was not discriminatory on its face, the fact that the company's workforce was drawn from an area with segregated schools that graduated significantly fewer African Americans than whites ultimately had an adverse impact on the ability of African Americans to move into higher-paying jobs. The decision established that such requirements had to have a business necessity, rather than just be a preference of the employer. The notion of disparate impact theory removed the necessity for the employee to prove any discriminatory intent.

Title VII's prohibition against discrimination on the basis of sex was also recognized by the courts hearing cases involving what is now recognized as sexual harassment. Initially, the courts focused on quid pro quo sexual harassment cases, in which the employer conditioned some aspect of employment, such as pay increases, promotions, and keeping one's job, on compliance with the sexual demands of the agent of the employer—such as supervisor, manager, or owner, and found that that such activity, although deplorable, did not represent a violation of Title VII. Unfortunately, not until 1986, did the U.S. Supreme Court, relying on EEOC guidelines on sexual harassment, find that the creation of a hostile work environment through overt acts of sexual harassment or through "discriminatory intimidation, ridicule, and insult, whether based on sex, race, religion, or national origin," violated Title VII. This decision established the "hostile work environment" theory of sexual harassment. It also helped to define later decisions establishing the liability of employers for the actions of supervisors and other employees.

In 1990, Congress enacted the ADA. This set of regulations prohibited discrimination in employment against those defined as "disabled," and it required that employers take steps under the concept of "reasonable accommodation" to eradicate barriers against applicants and current employees who under the law were defined as disabled. In 1993, Congress enacted the FMLA, which provided a new entitlement for employees. For eligible employees of covered employers, the FMLA provided 3 new entitlements: up to 12 weeks of unpaid leave for a variety of reasons, a guarantee of continuation of employer-paid health insurance during the period of leave, and a guarantee of a return to the same or similar position as the employee had left. It also created the concept of "intermittent leave," which allows an employee to take the unpaid leave in increments.

In 1998, the Court identified that same-sex sexual harassment was also covered under Title VII. But the Court also observed that the employer should be able to decrease liability in sexual harassment suits and so if the employer tried to prevent and correct such harassment—usually through the mechanism of a sexual harassment policy and a complaint procedure—and if the complaining party did not use the complaint procedure, the employer would be able to defend against liability for the supervisor's actions. This decision also covered other forms of harassment such as racial harassment. However, this defense would not hold if the complaining employee was terminated or was denied income.

STATUS OF EMPLOYMENT

Employment in the private sector generally consists of 2 possibilities: at-will employment and employment under a contract. The at-will doctrine allows employers to dismiss an employee at any time for any reason at all, be it good or bad. Also under this doctrine, employees have a corresponding right to leave employment at any time without notice or reason. This doctrine, however, does have restrictions. For example, states have restricted the freedom of employers to regulate legal, off-duty conduct. For example, the court held that terminating an employee for refusing to commit perjury violated the public policy of having all persons speak truthfully in court. Similarly, persons reporting violations of law (whistle-blowing) or reporting for jury duty are also covered. However, many of these restrictions are determined by individual states. The states may not loosen any federal law such as the Civil Rights Act of 1991 that prohibits an employer's ability to dismiss employees on the basis of sex, race, religion, national origin, color, age, or disability or in retaliation for exercising an employee's rights under those laws. Employment under a contract is sometimes used by employers. These contracts typically involve basic aspects of employment, such as salary, benefits, and work to be performed, and often provide for dismissal of the person for reasons such as misconduct. These contracts may also regulate activities beyond the period of the contract by invoking noncompetition clauses that limit the person's ability to work in the same or a similar field of work. However, "noncompete" clauses must be reasonable with respect to radius of restriction and some other elements.

Another area that is often the source of concern and confusion is the constitutionality of certain behaviors, specifically those covered by the First Amendment (free speech) and the Fourth Amendment (unlawful searches) of the U.S. Constitution. There is a clear dichotomy here. For instance, employers in the private sector have no obligation regarding the first and fourth amendments and can prohibit speech that the employer does not like and can conduct random drug tests of their employees in addition to rummaging through an employee's locked desk drawers, search secured lockers, and even go into an employees' locked cars. Employees working in the public/government sector can rely on these amendments, and the employer is unable to conduct any of the above activities that violate the Constitution and its amendments. Thus, constitutional protections are available only to government employees and not to employees working in the private sector.

EMPLOYEE RELATIONS

Employee relations, as an aspect of HRM, has evolved over the years. Successful HR professionals need a firm knowledge of both state and federal employment laws, in addition to the organization's own policies and practices. In reality, employee relations activities are potentially a part of every HR decision or plan in which an organization engages. From an HR point of view, organizational difficulties can be found in 3 areas:

- Decisions involving recruitment, selection, or job advancement
- Decisions involving discipline, termination, or both
- Ensuring organizational compliance with federal employment laws, such as the FLSA or the FMLA

An area of ongoing difficulty is in the selection process following the interview of potential candidates. There are increased worries about the "legal/illegal" questions such as "Are you pregnant?" "How old are you?" or "What religious holidays do you observe?" However, from a technical point of view, there is only one specifically prohibited question under federal employment law: "Are you disabled?" The ADAAA specifically prohibits asking applicants whether they have a disability or not. None of the other questions violate any specific provision of law. However, those questions are all high-risk questions for several reasons. For instance, none of those questions are job related or consistent with business necessity and may indicate an intent to discriminate, which could lead to EEOC scrutiny and violation. Other areas that are quite suspect are determining that a position must be exempt (not eligible for overtime) because the organization cannot afford to pay overtime; the policy that if compensatory time ("comp time") is not used then it is lost; and the belief that interns are volunteers and do not have to compensated.

The way a health care organization handles employee discipline can be critical because it may have more strategic weight than in other work environments, as work that is sloppy, careless, or negligent can have a significant impact on patient care, even to the point of fatality. In addition, poor customer service can have a significant impact on both revenue and reputation of the organization.

Some other issues related to employee relations but are also affected by employment law:

- Romance in the workplace—The workplace is an ideal place to meet other people. Both extremes have been identified, each with its own inherent problems. One extreme is the use of "love contracts" in which employees agree not to date colleagues or subordinates; the other extreme occurs when the employer encourages romance between coworkers.
- Employee privacy around health issues covered by the Health Insurance Portability and Accountability Act and other confidentiality issues often create confusion and stress.
- State employment and nondiscrimination laws sometimes have greater protections for employees or restrictions on employers than comparable federal laws and which vary from state to state. Thus, HR managers must know their own state's regulations.
- Pregnancy discrimination (including lactation discrimination)—Awareness of this issue was given new impetus by the lactation provisions in the Affordable Care Act.
- Drug testing for applicants and employees—This topic not only involves constitutional restrictions for government workers but also varies from state to state.
- Preemployment medical testing or "fitness for duty" testing—This aspect of the ADAAA has had significant impact in a variety of situations, especially in health care.

- Workers' compensation laws—These laws are generally state specific.
- Safety and health issues—This category includes the laws and regulations enforced by the Occupational Safety and Health Administration.

PROFESSIONALISM: HAVING KNOWLEDGE AND SKILLS

Dreyfus and Dreyfus (2009) contend that both theoretical knowledge and practiced response are needed in the acquisition of skill in a profession. They lay out 5 stages of abilities that an individual passes through as he or she develops a skill:

1. ***Novice.*** At this stage, the novice learns tasks and skills that enable him or her to determine actions based on recognized situations. Rules and guidelines direct the novice's energy and action at this stage.
2. ***Advanced beginner.*** At this stage, the advanced beginner has gained enough experience and knowledge that certain behaviors become automatic, and he or she can begin to learn when tasks should be addressed.
3. ***Competent.*** At this stage, the competent individual has mastered the practiced response of definable tasks and processes and has acquired the ability to deal with the unexpected events that may not conform to plans.
4. ***Proficient.*** At this stage, the proficient individual has developed the ability to discern a situation, intuitively assess it, plan what needs to be done, decide on an action, and perform the action with less effort than in the earlier stages.
5. ***Expert.*** At this stage, the expert can accomplish the goals without realizing that rules are being followed because the skill and knowledge required to reach the goal have become second nature.

HEALTH CARE PROFESSIONALS

As health care evolves, more professionals are needed who are empowered to make decisions without direct supervision, which requires an understanding of both theory and practice. Health care workers include professionals such as physicians, nurses, dentists, nurse practitioners, and physician assistants. Functional training teaches personnel to perform tasks but does not teach the theory behind the practice. These allied health care workers include technicians, licensed practical/vocational nurses, and certified nurse assistants. Health care workers are employed in a variety of settings, including hospitals, ambulatory care organizations, pharmaceutical companies, physicians' offices, and research institutes.

Health care managers organize, coordinate, and manage the delivery of health services; provide leadership; and guide the strategic direction of health care organizations. The variety and numbers of health care professionals they employ, the complexity of health care delivery, and environmental pressures to provide access, quality, and efficient services make health care institutions among the most complex organizations to manage.

SOME CONSIDERATIONS FOR HUMAN RESOURCE MANAGEMENT

The role of HRM in health care organizations is to develop and implement systems, in accordance with regulatory guidelines and licensure laws, for selection, evaluation, and retention of health care professionals. HR managers must understand that each profession and specialty has specific requirements for the individual to qualify for an entry-level position in his or her profession. In addition, requirements of oversight and monitoring agencies such as national accrediting organizations (e.g., TJC), regulatory bodies (e.g., Centers for Medicare and Medicaid Services), and licensure authorities (e.g., state licensing boards) should be considered in all aspects of HRM.

Some of the issues that the HR department must consider include the following:

- **Qualifications of staff**. When developing a comprehensive employee compensation program, qualifications for each position must be developed and stated in writing. The job description generally contains the level of education, experience, responsibilities, physical skills, and any specific certification or licensure requirements. The HR manager must be aware of the requirements for all health care workers.
- **Licensure and certifications**. The HR department must have a procedure for verifying active and unrestricted licenses before initial employment and also have a mechanism for tracking the expiration dates of licenses and certifications and ensuring license/certification renewal. In addition, a copy of each license and certification must be on file in the HR department.
- **Career ladders**. During the recruitment process, the HR manager must consider employment history, including the explanation of gaps in employment. Also, on an ongoing basis, evaluate the employee's progressive breadth and depth of responsibilities when considering promotion. These "career ladders" are often based on the Dreyfus and Dreyfus (2009, pp. 1–24) model of novice to expert, and experience may be used as a criterion for promotion.
- **Educational services**. Every health care organization should provide an orientation for all new employees, which should include the mission, vision,

and value. Health care professionals require continual lifelong learning. Health care organizations should have internal and external training and development plans to ensure professionals achieve competency in new technologies, programs, and equipment and are aware of policy, procedure, and protocol changes. Many licensure and regulatory agencies require certain competencies to be renewed—usually annually—in areas such as cardiopulmonary resuscitation, safety and infection control, disaster planning, and confidentiality.

- **Practitioner impairment**. Health care professionals are accountable to the public for maintaining high professional standards. The governing body of the organization is ultimately responsible for the quality of care rendered, which is easily jeopardized by an impaired practitioner. An impaired practitioner is a health care professional who is unable to carry out his or her professional duties with reasonable skill and safety because of a physical or mental illness, including deterioration through aging, loss of motor skill, or excessive use of drugs and alcohol. HR managers must have policies and procedures in place to regularly evaluate the performance of all health care professionals to ensure their competence and proficiency. Mechanisms to identify and deal with the impaired practitioner must be in place. Every state licensing authority maintains legal requirements for reporting impaired practitioners.
- **Workforce diversity**. Workforce composition now and in the future requires continuing to monitor and encourage diversity within the health care professions. Although workforce diversity is a broad concept, it focuses on differences in gender, age, race, and sexual orientation. It is apparent that some professions are dominated by one gender or the other as demonstrated by the predominantly female field of nursing or the historically predominantly male field of health care management. Ultimately, the diversity of the members of a profession should ideally reflect the diversity of the members of the population being served.

UNIONS, UNIONIZATION, AND MANAGING THE RELATIONSHIPS

The National Labor Relations Act (NLRA) governs the labor-management relations of business firms and organizations. The National Labor Relations Board is responsible for administering and enforcing the NLRA. This board provides procedures through which employees can choose a union as a collective bargaining representative. In 1974, an amendment designating procedures that limit strikes in health care organizations was added to the NLRA. The amendment requires a 10-day strike notice, allows the National Labor Relations Board to determine the legality of the strike, and gives the organization time to put in place provisions to protect the level of patient care. Labor rights include the right to organize and bargain collectively, solicit and distribute union information, picket, and strike. Management rights include the right to receive a strike notice, hire replacement workers, restrict union activity to prescribed areas, prohibit union activity during working hours, and prohibit unionization of supervisors (Pozgar, 2016).

A union (also known as "organized labor") is an organization formed by employees for the purpose of acting as a single unit when dealing with management about workplace issues. The union is the exclusive bargaining agent for the employees. Because employees must authorize a union to represent them, unions are not present in every organization. Unions are typically viewed as threats by management because they interfere with management's ability to make and implement decisions that affect employees so that once the union is present, management can no longer unilaterally make decisions about the terms and conditions of work. Instead, management must negotiate these decisions with the union. Also, employees can no longer communicate directly with management about work issues but instead must go through the union. In this scenario, the union acts as a "middleman" between the employee and management; the union is relatively expensive for both parties to maintain, which is why employers have a strong incentive to keep unions out of the organization. Once it is apparent that a union will be in place, it is important to develop strategies and goals to implement a positive labor relations program. This requires an understanding of the generic labor relations process of organizing, negotiating, and administering contracts with the union. Because of the historical adversarial nature of the relationship, to promote a productive and positive labor-management partnership, compromise by both parties is necessary. Although both parties have a vested interest in the success and survival of the organization, each party's goals are quite different. The union will look to improve the employee's salary, benefit, and work structure package, whereas management's interest is in containing costs and quality improvement. Thus, the challenge for management is working with the union to reconcile differences in a fair and consistent manner.

The desire to unionize is believed to result from 3 issues: wages, benefits, and employee perceptions about the workplace. Thus, management must rely on monitoring the ongoing, negative signals or indicators in the workplace. Some of the behaviors that may indicate organizing activities or the potential for organizing employees include the following:

- **Increased employee turnover—especially to competitors.** Although turnover in health care organizations is traditionally higher than in other organizations, if employees are moving at a higher-than-normal rate to competing organizations in the local area, this may indicate dissatisfaction rather than career opportunities.
- **Increased employee-generated incidents.** This includes horizontal violence, theft or damage of the organization's property, and/or an increasing level of insubordination.
- **Increase in the number of grievances.** More grievances are being filed with the HR department compared with informal settlements of supervisors and employees.
- **Decrease in communication.** Employees seem reluctant to provide feedback and generally become quiet when managers enter the room.
- **Increase in off-site meetings.** It seems that staff are congregating more at off-site locations.
- **Increase in grapevine activity.** Rumors increase in number and intensity.
- **Increase in absenteeism or lateness.** The potential exists that employees are engaging in union-organizing activities before and during work hours.
- **Increase in negative social media activity.** Postings on Facebook and other social networking Web sites espouse negativity regarding the workplace and management.

SUMMARY

Despite all the changes seen in the provision of health care, people continue to play a critical and central role in providing health services. Automation and other technologic advances have allowed other industries to downsize, whereas technologic changes in the health care industry generate the need for highly trained and well-managed health professionals. Other industries have outsourced an incalculable number of jobs, whereas health care services cannot be significantly outsourced. Moreover, the health care workforce is under increasing pressure. Incentive structures have led to increased severity among hospitalized patients, and cost containment pressures have led in some instances to decreases in staffing, with the remaining workers facing an increased workload. Managers are being asked to manage and retain a workforce that in many cases are highly stressed. Effective job design, training, and performance management mechanisms need to be well developed and executed effectively (Fried & Fottler, 2015).

QUESTIONS

1. An important area where the HR department is tasked is:
   a. Acting as legal counsel for employees
   b. Providing financial advice to employees
   c. Instilling motivation for optimal employee satisfaction
   d. Assisting employees in finding work outside the organization
2. The use of self-managed teams and decentralization:
   a. Are required in a union environment
   b. Minimize management layers
   c. Are often problematic for managers and staff alike
   d. Are a form of shared governance
3. The HR model of conflict is which one of the following?
   a. Conflict must be avoided
   b. Conflict is a natural and inevitable outcome in any group
   c. Conflict should be encouraged
   d. Conflict indicates malfunctioning within the group
4. Characteristics of health care organizations that drive exceptional outcomes in patient experience, engagement, and quality of care include all of the following except:
   a. Ensuring a focused and rigid culture
   b. Promoting solid patient-staff relationships
   c. Selecting appropriate fit of staff to the organization
   d. Maintaining a central focus on customer service
5. When identifying screening indicators that could result in poor clinical outcomes, the organization will need to identify all of the following except:
   a. Thresholds for acceptable levels
   b. Benchmarks for the industry
   c. Root cause analysis of issues
   d. Problematic personnel
6. The statute that covers employment for persons older than 39 years is the:
   a. ADA
   b. ADEA
   c. FLSA
   d. FMLA
7. Which of the following statements about unionization is false?
   a. Unions are typically viewed as threats by management.
   b. Employees must authorize a union to represent them.
   c. Management has limited decision-making authority about the terms and conditions of work.
   d. Employers cannot communicate directly with employees about work issues.

ANSWERS: 1-c, 2-b, 3-b, 4-a, 5-d, 6-b, 7-c

References

Dreyfus, H. L., & Dreyfus, S. E. (2009). The relationship of theory and practice in the acquisition of skill. In Benner, P., Tanner C. A., & Chesla, C. A. (Eds.), *Expertise in nursing practice: Caring, clinical judgment and ethics* (2nd ed.). New York: Springer.

Equal Employment Opportunity Commission. (2014). *Title VII of the civil rights act of 1964*. Retrieved from www.eeoc.gov/laws/statutes/titlevii.cfm.

Fried, B. J., & Fottler, M. D. (Eds.). (2015). *Human resources in healthcare: Managing for success* (4th ed.). Chicago: Health Administration Press.

Gomez-Mejia, L. R., Balkin, D. B., & Cardy, R. L. (2012). *Managing human resources* (7th ed.). Upper Saddle River, NJ: Pearson Education.

Platonova, E. A., & Hernandez, S. R. (2013). Innovative human resource practices in U.S. hospitals: An empirical study. *Journal of Healthcare Management, 58*(4), 290–301.

Pozgar, G. (2016). *Legal aspects of health care administration* (12th ed.). Burlington, MA: Jones & Bartlett.

Society for Human Resource Management. (2012). *Challenges facing HR over the next 10 years*. Retrieved from www.shrm.org/research/surveyfindings/articles/pages/challenges-facinghroverthenext10years.aspx.

Society for Human Resource Management. (2014). *Future insights: The top trends for 2014 according to SHRM's HR subject matter expert panels*. Retrieved from www.shrm.org/research/futureworkplacetrends/pages/toptrendsfor2014.aspx.

Wolf, J. A. (2012). *Organizational culture: A critical choice at the heart of an exceptional patient experience*. The Beryl Institute. Retrieved from www.theberylinstitute.org.

CHAPTER

7

Cultural and Intergenerational Diversity

Virginia "Ginny" Wilson

This chapter will review:

CULTURAL DIVERSITY

LEADER COMPETENCIES IN CULTURAL DIVERSITY

GENERATIONAL DIVERSITY

GENERATIONAL TRAITS

LEVERAGING CULTURAL AND GENERATIONAL DIVERSITY

CULTURE AND CULTURAL DIVERSITY

Culture is defined as a set of practices among a group of individuals, the norms that set the standards. Cultural diversity is a difference from the social standards and interactions of another group (Alpert, 2018; Leininger & McFarland, 2006). It is the differences in cultures, the diversity that enriches organizations and supports a mission of serving all.

A workforce with cultural diversity brings new ideas, new problem-solving methods, and new ways of doing that enriches the organization and the marketplace it serves. The literature supports the benefits of a culturally diverse workforce that for health care organizations results not only in business success but also in improved quality and safety, and nurse and patient satisfaction (Dudas, 2012; Lowe & Archibald, 2009). Lowe (1994) argues that cultural competence in nursing is the use of culture-specific behaviors, actions, and interventions that are unique to the culture, a competence that would apply to leadership as well. Because the business of health care is service delivery, having a culturally competent workforce enhances the outcomes of the organization.

Leaders are responsible in a culturally diverse workplace and marketplace to continually improve their own cultural awareness and sensitivity. In doing so, they will be better equipped to leverage the diversity in the workforce supporting recruitment, hiring, and retention activities. The American Organization of Nurse Executives supports diversity in the workplace and extends diversity as a competency for all nurse leaders (AONE, 2015):

- Establish an environment that values diversity (e.g., age, gender, race, religion, ethnicity, sexual orientation, culture).
- Establish cultural competency in the workforce.
- Incorporate cultural beliefs into care delivery.
- Provide an environment conducive to opinion sharing, exploration of ideas, and achievement of outcomes.

Cultural competency is an awareness, an attitude, and behaviors that enhance communication between diverse cultural groups supporting a diverse workplace and populations served (Dudas, 2012; Mareno & Hart, 2014). Developing cultural competence and embracing cultural diversity is a leadership expectation that maximizes all human capital and potential in an organization and leverages that diversity into an organization better positioned to care for all groups. Recognizing that health care organizations serve diverse individuals, a culturally competent and diverse workforce can serve increasingly diverse customers and meet the challenges of an increasingly complex health care delivery business environment.

GENERATIONAL DIVERSITY

The topic of generational diversity, the dynamics of the workforce, and the impact on organizations are as important as cultural diversity in the discussion of leadership and organizational success. Although each generation is defined by the social events of the time, the political climate of the era, and the impact on growing minds, it is important to remember that stereotyping each individual hinders the ability to maximize the human capital that each member of the workforce team brings to the organization. To prepare for those crucial conversations, to capitalize on individual strengths that contribute to the success and stability of the organization, and to create an engaged and satisfied workforce, it is necessary to have a working knowledge of the strengths and challenges of the 4 generations that currently make up the workforce.

Research on generational diversity is not new. An early definition of generational diversity can be attributed to Mannheim (1953) who described generations as a group of individuals born within the same time span and affected by the same historical and social context. The definitions discussed in the contemporary literature include 4 age groups now in the workforce together defining the generations within years of birth (Crampton & Hodge, 2007; Lyons, 2005; McGuire, Todnem By, & Hutchings, 2007; Merrill, 2008; Trunk, 2007). The Matures or the Silent Generation, the Baby boomers, the Generation X, and the Millennials or Generation Y make up the current workforce with a note that Generation Z is on the horizon to join the workforce (Knoll, 2014).

The Mature workforce born from 1920 to 1946 make up 3% of the workforce today (Bennett, 2017). Although many are 70 years and older and have retired from the workplace, there are still many who choose to stay on and work in senior (leadership and management) roles even in a part-time status. This group of individuals grew up in lean times, the Great Depression and austerity, was exposed to major international conflicts, World War II and the Korean conflict, and as a result considers work a privilege. Their work ethic includes hard work, carving one's own path, and contributing to the long-term success of their organizations. This is not a group formed from a culture of immediate gratification (Ferri-Reed, 2013) but a group that believes in productivity and effort leading to advancement and promotion. They are loyal, respectful of authority, reliable, and consistent. Their challenges lie in having to learn and embrace technology, which they will do, but they expect to be respected for their experience. One-on-one communication is a skill they excel in, and they do well in interpersonal and team environments (Duchscher & Cowin, 2004). Communication is personal and written; no matter the delivery method, Matures prefer formal communication.

Baby boomers born from 1946 to 1964 make up a large percentage of the current workforce, with at least 49% of them working full-time or part-time (Harter & Agrawal, 2014). This generation reports that 31% of them plan to work beyond the retirement age of 67 years, which translates into retaining intellectual capital in the workforce on a full-time or part-time status depending on personal health and financial issues (Newport, 2015). They grew up in an era of social change and as such are open to change, growth, and rules that change (Crampton & Hodge, 2007; Lyons, 2005; Trunk, 2007). Baby boomers are known to be loyal, value success, employ a strong work ethic, and commit to a cause they believe in. Their challenges lie in expecting all members of the work team to embrace a "workaholic" attitude, being judgmental when disagreed with, and being somewhat self-centered. Baby boomers communicate well face to face, monitor body language, but have embraced technology and have learned to include social media communication techniques as well.

Generation X members born from 1965 to 1980 have surpassed the Baby boomer workforce in numbers only to be eclipsed by Millennial workforce numbers in 2015 (Fry, 2011). They grew up in an era when the status quo no longer existed. There was the fall of the Berlin Wall, Watergate, the energy crisis, and age of gender definition such as women's liberation. They prefer flexibility, are creative, want work to be fun, can be skeptical, and question authority (Crampton & Hodge, 2007; The National Oceanographic and Atmospheric Association Office of Diversity, 2006). Their challenges lie in a desire to be self-sufficient and autonomous yet needing immediate feedback and reassurance that what they are doing is valued. This generation is not necessarily loyal to employers but is loyal to their family and friends (Karp, Fuller, & Sirias, 2002; The National Oceanographic and Atmospheric Association Office of Diversity, 2006). Their communication style is direct, and it is necessary to keep things short, simple, and to the point to maintain attention. Generation X grew up with technology and gaming consoles and are used to technology, so they communicate using email and social media formats.

Millennial generation members born from 1980 to the late 1990s have surpassed the Generation X workforce in numbers in 2015 (Fry, 2011). They grew up in an era of being connected, closer family units, social media, Internet access, and portable computing and were influenced by 9/11 and Oklahoma City and school shootings, which helped form their conservative value sets. They are entrepreneurial and goal oriented and enjoy multitasking and want to know their work is meaningful, so like Generation X, they need continual feedback to validate their contribution. Millennials tend to be optimistic, value team work, and embrace diversity (The National Oceanographic and Atmospheric Association Office of Diversity, 2006). Their challenges include a sense of entitlement for on-demand information, work to acquire money to be spent on personal choices, and exciting/challenging work that is not routine. They prefer to communicate using technology: email, voice mail, social media, and other short forms of messaging (Table 7.1).

THE ORGANIZATION AND GENERATIONAL DIVERSITY

Success of the organization depends on communication among and between all members of the workforce. Because communication is the life blood of any organization, an interruption or disruption of information will have

TABLE 7.1 Generational Traits

	Matures	Baby Boomers	Generation X	Millennials
Traits	Conservative Loyal Patriotic	Idealistic Loyal Want to please Politically correct	Pragmatic Self-sufficient Adaptability Creative	Confident Self-sufficient Social orientation
Communication	Face to face	Telephone	Email	Instant messaging/text
Work ethic	Dedicated/loyal	Driven	Balance	Eager but anxious
Work is	On the clock	Important	Will it matter if I get it done?	Am I done yet?
In the workplace	Being needed beyond retirement age	Recognition	Information/reassurance	Praise/reassurance/challenged/fun

Drawn from the academic and popular articles consulted and referenced.

a distinct impact on the organization's function. According to Legas and Sims (2011), productivity and transmission of critical information from the experienced workforce to new or less experienced workers is critical. Yet, communication disruption often results from generational differences and misinterpretation. Hanna (2009) argues that because each generation learns and interacts differently, the success of an organization with 4 generations of employees depends on effective communication. The Mature and Baby boomers, those with the most work experience, need to communicate effectively with the Generation X and Millennials. This helps to ensure that the team workforce effort and organization benefit from interpersonal communications to avoid dysfunction and decreased morale (Dudas, 2012; Legas & Sims, 2011).

Organizational success is measured by sustainability and profitability (Collins, 2001) and is achieved through the cycle of input, process, and output. The generations view the elements of the cycle in a different manner, so recognizing and optimizing the strength of each generation contributes to the success of the organization through work activities (Tolbize, 2008). Matures and Baby boomers are the strength to the process elements, whereas Generation X and Millennials focus on the outcomes element. A leader's role is to optimize open lines of communication and work opportunities to make the input, process, and outcome cycle flow smoothly.

OPPORTUNITIES TO IMPROVE LOYALTY ACROSS GENERATIONS

Generational diversity is thought to contribute to turnover rates and loyalty. Although the general belief is that Generation X is the least loyal, Deal (2007) argues that loyalty may be a result of factors other than the generation, such as age or other factors. Could the lack of advancement opportunities for Generation X and Millennials influence the length of employment at an organization? According to Legas and Sims (2011), Baby boomers are delaying retirement, remaining in organizations in leadership and management positions, and preventing the possibility of upward mobility for generations following them. The fact that there is no restriction on hours worked and social security payments when an individual has reached full retirement age (Harter & Agrawal, 2014; Social Security Administration, 2017) may contribute to the ongoing outward mobility of Generation X and Millennials to secure upwardly mobile positions in organizations in the continued future.

Organizations will need to improve opportunities to retain young talent through a series of activities that include opportunities to learn new skills, leadership and professional development, opportunities for advancement or leadership roles, mentorship, and better compensation in the form of benefits and salary (Deal, 2007; Legas & Sims, 2011). Knowledge and skill development are viewed by Generation X and Millennials as a means to versatility (The Center for Generational Differences, 2010) and as such should be key foundational pieces to developing a culture of continuous learning in an organization that values generational diversity. Because the Matures and Baby boomers will be a part of organizations for the foreseeable future, what they know and can convey to upcoming talent should not be ignored but transformed into a learning environment that all generations can benefit from (Gallup, 2016; Legas & Sims, 2011; The Center for Generational Differences, 2010; Tolbize, 2008).

LEVERAGING GENERATIONAL DIVERSITY

For organizations to leverage generational diversity to their advantage, it is now the time to recognize the value in 4 generations working together and to strengthen those working relationships for the good of the organization. The conflicts, they may be referred to as clashpoints, that occur are a result of misunderstanding and miscommunication that result in a reactionary approach to generational diversity instead of a proactive one (Deal, 2007; Lancaster & Stillman, 2002; Legas & Sims, 2011; McGuire et al., 2007; The Center for Generational Differences, 2010). Recognizing the strengths and challenges of each generation can be the foundation to developing programs that will be beneficial to all, promote open lines of communication, and support the organization's goals in the marketplace.

VALUE OF GENERATIONAL DIVERSITY TRAINING

Diversity training can be that program that explores and exposes each generation to the strength and challenges of the others. Just as in the case of cultural diversity, the benefit of generational diversity lies in the recognition that everyone is not created the same, that even within the generations there are subcultures, and that learning about each other contributes to understanding differences and beliefs (Bennett, 2017; Gibson, Greenwood, & Murphy, 2009; Legas and Sims, 2011; McGuire et al., 2007; The Center for Generational

Differences, 2010). However, as Legas and Sims (2011) argue, the lack of evaluation of current diversity training programs creates the question of what is working? In a discipline that focuses heavily on evidence-informed practice, the need for research on existing generational diversity training programs outcomes is seen as important to creating the programs that will work based on organization's generational makeup.

Diversity training can also be viewed as a value added for the marketplace. In the case of patient care delivery systems, generational diversity training can provide a better understanding of not only the pathology that requires care but also the care based on communicating and caring in a style that respects and speaks to the age group of the patient (DeVoe, Wallace, & Fryer, 2009a, 2009b). Communication does play an important role in health care delivery and outcomes. As such "communication could be useful to design practice-level interventions that enhance services and also to develop national policies that improve health care delivery and health outcomes" (DeVoe et al., 2009b, p. 126), which could be accomplished in a generational diversity training program.

Organizations to date have focused on cultural and gendered diversity training but are in their infancy stages of making generational diversity training a core component that benefits the organization, the workforce, and the marketplace. Until formal programs can be developed along the lines of established successes, a complementary approach for bridging the gap in the present is suggested in a formal mentor program.

MENTORSHIP ACROSS THE GENERATIONS

Mentoring between the generations provides an opportunity to leverage generational diversity in an ongoing manner. Because mentoring includes communication, observation, and receiving feedback, there is an opportunity for workforce generations to get to know each other better and not just in a line authority relationship. As a process, each side of the mentoring relationship can learn from each other in a relationship that lasts more than one encounter. Subsequently, mentoring is two sided, self-reflective, and a method for information exchange by which a multigenerational workforce can learn from each other without authority overlays and generational bias (Schlimbach, 2010; The Center for Generational Diversity, 2010).

Mentoring recognizes the wealth of knowledge gained over a lifetime of experience for the Traditionalists and Baby boomers and supports Generation X and

Millennials by providing feedback, coaching, and professional development. Mentoring may take place in the traditional one-on-one manner, but there is evidence to suggest that e-mentoring also helps fill the need and is welcomed by Generation X and Millennials (Fry, 2011; Pietsch & Williamson, 2010). The key to successful mentoring, face to face or using technology, is to have organizational support and the time and resources to do so (Posey-Goodwin, 2013; Yamamura & Stedham, 2007).

LEADERSHIP IMPLICATIONS

Leaders have the primary role of understanding generational diversity and bridging the gaps. Creating a harmonious, productive work environment is as important as knowledge transfer from experienced employees to newer employees. This can only be accomplished when there is respect and communication that works among the differing generations. Profit and positive margins are about the success of an organization (Collins, 2001), but it is the people themselves who must be invested in to support retention, not turn over, in an environment of acceptance and understanding (Fry, 2011; Legas and Sims, 2011; McGuire et al., 2007; The Center for Generational Differences, 2010).

Providing the resources for generational diversity and mentoring programs is a necessity, not a luxury. To avoid an environment full of clashpoints (Lancaster & Stillman, 2002), a leader's role must include building a workforce culture that helps knowing each other, understands the differences, can communicate effectively, and respect that one size does not fit all (Fry, 2011; Karp et al., 2002; Sherman, 2006; Wilson & Foltz, 2005). That can be accomplished only with a leader's action plan and budget that supports education, coaching, mentoring, and capitalizing of generational differences to strengthen the environment.

CONCLUSION

Diversity, defined "the state of being diverse or a variety" (Oxford Dictionaries, 2017), has lent itself to organizations focusing on cultural-gender-sexual orientation and now generational diversity. The collective focus is on the recognition that the sum of an organization results from many parts, each different, but important in the work toward a collective goal of meeting the organization's goals. By embracing diversity, an organization is capable of leveraging that diversity and linking the workforce, the workplace, and the marketplace together.

QUESTIONS

1. A primary leadership behavior that improves intergenerational cooperation is:
   a. Use of social media
   b. Staff meetings
   c. Company billboards
   d. Communication
2. Developing a multicultural workforce that represents many groups and backgrounds is referred to as:
   a. Hiring resources
   b. Social agenda
   c. Leveraging diversity
   d. Affirmative action
3. The generation most noted for their use and understanding of technology is:
   a. Generation X
   b. Baby boomers
   c. Matures
   d. Millennials
4. Cultural diversity in an organization enriches an organization and:
   a. Meets state and federal laws
   b. Supports a mission of serving all
   c. Is required by the Equal Employment Opportunities Commission
   d. Brings in new customers
5. The workforce of the future is predicted to continue to include which generation that will not have hours of work limited by Social Security restrictions?
   a. Generation X
   b. Millennials
   c. Baby boomers
   d. Generation Z
6. In work activities which two groups excel in the outcomes element of a cycle?
   a. Matures and Millennials
   b. Baby boomers and Generation X
   c. Generation X and Matures
   d. Generation X and Millennials

ANSWERS: 1-d, 2-c, 3-d, 4-b, 5-c, 6-d

References

American Organization of Nurse Executives. (2015). *AONE nurse executive competencies.* Chicago, IL: American Organization of Nurse Executives.

Alpert R. (2018). Cultural diversity in the workplace. *Diversity resources.* Retrieved from https://www.diversityresources.com/cultural-diversity-workplace/.

Bennett, M. (2017). *A formal introduction to the five generations of employees in your workforce. Ethics and compliance matters.* NavexGlobal. Retrieved from http://www.navexglobal.com/blog/formal-introduction-five-generations-employees-your-workforce.

Collins, J. (2001). *Good to great.* New York, NY: Harper Business.

Crampton, S. M., & Hodge, J. W. (2007). Generations in the workplace: Understanding age diversity. *The Business Review, Cambridge*, *9*(1), 16–23.

Deal, J. (2007). *Retiring the generation gap: How the young and old can find common ground.* Jossey-Bass.

DeVoe, J. E., Wallace, L. S., & Fryer, G. E. (2009a). Measuring patients' perceptions of communication with healthcare providers: Do differences in demographic and socioeconomic characteristics matter? *Health Expectations*, *12*(1), 70–80.

DeVoe, J. E., Wallace, L. S., & Fryer, G. E. (2009b). Patient age influences perceptions about health care communication. *Family Medicine*, *41*(2), 126–133.

Duchscher, J. E., & Cowin, L. (2004). Multigenerational nurses in the workplace. *Journal of Nursing Administration*, *34*(11), 493–501.

Dudas, K. I. (2012). Cultural competence: An evolutionary concept analysis. *Nursing Education Perspectives*, *33*(5), 317–321. Retrieved from https://www.library.drexel.edu/cgi-bin/r.cgi/login?url=https://search-proquest-com.ezproxy2.library.drexel.edu/docview/1086347577?accountid=10559.

Ferri-Reed, J. (January 2013). Quality,conflict and communication across the generations. *Journal for Quality and Participation; Cincinnati*, *35.4*, 12–14.

Fry, B. (2011). *A nurse's guide to intergenerational diversity*. Canadian Federation of Nurses Unions. Retrieved from http://neltoolkit.rnao.ca/sites/default/files/CFNU%20Thriving%20in%20Workplace.%20A%20Nurses%20Guide%20to%20Intergenerational%20Diversity.pdf.

Gibson, J. W., Greenwood, R. A., & Murphy Jr, E. F. (2009). Generational differences in the workplace: Personal values, behaviors, and popular beliefs. *Journal of Diversity Management*, *4*(3), 1.

Hanna, E. (May 1, 2009). New tactics needed to train Gen Y workers. *Hotel & Motel Management*, *224*(3), 1, 41. Retrieved from http://www.hotelworldnetwork.com/training/new-tactics-needed-train-gen-y.

Harter, J., & Agrawal, S. (2014). *Many baby boomers reluctant to retire. Economy*, Gallup. Retrieved from http://www.gallup.com/poll/166952/baby-boomers-reluctant-retire.aspx.

Karp, H., Fuller, C., & Sirias, D. (2002). *Bridging the boomer Xer gap: Creating authentic teams for high performance at work.* Palo Alto, CA: Davies-Black Publishing.

Knoll. (2014). *What comes after Y? Generation Z: Arriving to the office soon*. Retrieved from https://www.knoll.com/media/340/742/Infographic_Generation_Z_3pgs.pdf.

Lancaster, L. C., & Stillman, D. (2002). *When generations collide*. New York, NY: Harper Collins.

Legas M., & Sims C. (2011). Leveraging generational diversity in today's workplace. *Online Journal for Workforce Education and Development*, 5(3).

Leininger, M., & McFarland, M. (2006). *Cultural care diversity and universality: A worldwide nursing theory* (2nd ed.). Sudbury, MA: Jones and Bartlett.

Lowe, J. (1994). Developing cultural competence. *Florida Nurse*, *42*(2), 16.

Lowe, J., & Archibald, C. (2009). Cultural diversity: The intention of nursing. *Nursing Forum*, *44*(1),11–18.Retrievedfromhttps://www.library.drexel.edu/cgi-bin/r.cgi/login?url=https://search-proquest-com.ezproxy2.library.drexel.edu/docview/195004089?accountid=10559.

Lyons, S. (November 2005). Are gender differences in basic human values a generational phenomenon? *Sex Roles*, *53*,763–778. Retrieved from http://wwwfindarticles.com/p/articles/mi_m2294/is_9-10_53/ai_n16084047/print.

Mannheim, K. (1953). *Essays on sociology and social psychology*. New York, NY: Oxford University Press.

Mareno, N., & Hart, P. L. (2014). Cultural competency among nurses with undergraduate and graduate degrees: Implications for nursing education. *Nursing Education Perspectives*, *35*(2), 83–88. Retrieved from https://www.library.drexel.edu/cgi-bin/r.cgi/login?url=https://search-proquest-com.ezproxy2.library.drexel.edu/docview/1510501067?accountid=10559.

McGuire, D., Todnem By, R., & Hutchings, K. (2007). Towards a model of human resource solutions for achieving intergenerational interaction in organisations. *Journal of European Industrial Training, 31*(8), 592–608.

Merrill, D. (May 2008). Boomers pass the workplace torch. *The Lane Report, 23*(5), 34+.

Newport F. (2015). Only one third of the oldest baby boomers in the U.S. still working. *Economy: Gallup*. Retrieved from http://news.gallup.com/poll/181292/third-oldest-baby-boomers-working.aspx.

Oxford Dictionaries. (2017). Retrieved from https://www.oxforddictionaries.com/.

Pietsch M., & Williamson J. (2010). "Getting the pieces together": Negotiating the transition from pre-service to in-service teacher. *Asia-Pacific Journal of Teacher Education*, 38(4), 331–344.

Posey-Goodwin, P. (2013). *Exploring preferences of mentoring activities among generational groups of registered nurses in Florida (Order No. 3558212)*. Available from ProQuest Dissertations & Theses Global. (1350631029). Retrieved from https://www.library.drexel.edu/cgi-bin/r.cgi/login?url=https://search-proquest-com.ezproxy2.library.drexel.edu/docview/1350631029?accountid=10559.

Schlimbach, T. (2010). Intergenerational mentoring in Germany: Older people support young people's transitions from school to work. *Working with Older People: Community Care Policy & Practice, 14*(4), 4–15. Retrieved from EBSCOhost.

Sherman, R. (May 31, 2006). Leading a multigenerational nursing workforce: Issues, challenges and strategies. *OJIN: The Online Journal of Issues in Nursing, 11*(2), 3.

Social Security Administration. (2017). *Frequently asked questions*. Retrieved from https://faq.ssa.gov/link/portal/34011/34019/Article/3739/What-happens-if-I-work-and-get-Social-Security-retirement-benefits.

The Center for Generational Diversity. (2010). *Knowledge transfer and the emerging generations*. Common Sense Enterprises. Retrieved from https://commonsenseenterprises.net/wp-content/uploads/2015/11/knowledge_transfer_ebook.pdf.

The National Oceanographic and Atmospheric Association Office of Diversity. (2006). *Tips to improve the interaction among the generations: Traditionalists, boomers, X'ers and nexters*. Retrieved from http://honolulu.hawaii.edu/intranet/committees/FacDevCom/guidebk/teachtip/intergencomm.htm.

Tolbize A. (2008). Generational differences in the workplace. *Research and Training Center of Community Living*, 19, 1–13.

Trunk, P. (2007). *What generation Y really wants—Time*. Retrieved from http://www.time.com/time/magazine/article/0, 9171, 1640395,00.htm.

Wilson, C., & Foltz, J. (2005). Managing multiple generations at work. *Feed and Grain, 44*, 54–61. Retrieved from https://www.library.drexel.edu/cgi-bin/r.cgi/login?url=https://search-proquest-com.ezproxy2.library.drexel.edu/docview/197740557?accountid=10559.

Yamamura, J. H., & Stedham, Y. (2007). Meeting the information needs of professional staff. *The CPA Journal, 77*(10), 66–69.

CHAPTER

8

Ethics in Health Care and Nursing

Al Rundio

This chapter will review:

ETHICAL ISSUES

ETHICAL THEORIES

AN ETHICAL MODEL OF PRACTICE

LANDMARK ETHICAL CASES

ETHICS CASE STUDY

LEGAL ISSUES

LEGAL THEORIES

ANATOMY OF A MALPRACTICE CASE

CONTRACTS AND CONSENTS

This chapter discusses ethical and legal issues in health care and nursing: ethical theories, landmark ethical cases, and moral distress. Moral distress is defined as the following: "Moral distress is the pain or anguish affecting the mind, body or relationships to a situation in which the person is aware of the moral problem, acknowledges moral responsibility and makes a moral judgment about the correct action; yet as a result of real or perceived constraints, participates in perceived moral wrongdoing."

Each one of us has a moral compass. Obstacles may be internal or external. Acting in a manner contrary to personal and professional values undermines the individual's integrity and authenticity. It can cause painful feelings as well as psychological disequilibrium.

Areas of moral distress include the following:

- Clinical practice
- Management/administrative practice

- Research practice
- Personal situations

One should take a moral inventory of oneself and consider how often one has experienced moral distress in his or her professional role. This can be done daily, weekly, or monthly.

One should contemplate a situation in which one has experienced moral distress. Take notice of the physical sensations, feelings, and thoughts that arise.

The reality is that in health care today there are going to be times when our moral compass is challenged. We need to be ready to address these situations.

There is an interrelationship between ethics, laws, and morals. According to the American Nurses Association the ethical premise for nursing practice is that nurses help people regain and maintain health, help patients achieve a maximum potential, and help the dying patient (ANA, 2015).

The following ethical principles are critical to understand decision making in the field of ethics.

AUTONOMY

Autonomy is the freedom to be self-regulating (Guido, 2013). It is the primary objective in the provision of patient care. Autonomy is a patient right as long as what the patient wants is both legal and ethical. The person must be of sound mind.

FIDELITY

Fidelity is the duty to be faithful and loyal and to honor promises made. Having a nursing license is to honor promises made to the state through our laws, nursing boards and professional organizations through our standards and code of ethics. Accountability is based on fidelity. Ethical dilemmas result when nurses' duty requires loyalty to 2 opposite interests; they are accountable to themselves and they are also accountable to the clients that they serve.

JUSTICE

Duty dictates that there be equitable access and care to everyone who seeks health care. There are 2 forms of justice.

The first form is distributive justice. This is based on organizational and governmental decisions as to who gets what in the form of goods and services. One example is that all American citizens get covered with a universal form of health care.

The second form of justice is procedural justice. This is based on clear and known processes within distributive justice. In other words, if we are providing all American citizens with the universal form of health care coverage, exactly what is that coverage and how does this get implemented and distributed?

BENEFICENCE

This is the duty to be a patient advocate, that is, do good for a patient. Society believes strongly that a nurse will do good for a patient and also prevent harm or evil to the patient. This is an ethical principle that sometimes causes great angst for nurses.

NONMALEFICENCE

This is the duty to protect the patient from harm, that is, provide care without intentional or unintentional harm. This also implies protection of those who cannot protect themselves. It is the duty to prevent experiments that could harm the patient or unnecessary procedures done strictly as learning experiences.

VERACITY

Veracity is truthfulness. Truth is viewed as the cornerstone of nursing practice. It is both legal and ethical. It is not absolute in cases in which telling a client everything could cause additional harm to the patient. Nursing is known for its veracity and is the most trusted profession. In Gallup polls for several years nursing has been rated as number one for the most trusted profession secondary to veracity. The only year that nursing was not rated at this level was during the 9/11 attack, when New York firefighters were rated number one for veracity.

These 6 principles are critical to consider when rendering patient care and making ethical decisions.

Nurse administrators must be committed to the creation of an ethical practice environment. We must be committed to the client, to ourselves, and to our staff. We have a duty to support such an environment, and by doing so we also contribute to the profession of nursing.

OTHER THEORIES

Act Utilitarianism (Teleologic)

The focus is on the consequence of the actions. The approach here is to do good or to provide the greatest amount of happiness for the greatest number of people or the least amount of harm to the greatest number of people.

An example of this theory is mandatory vaccinations for all children who attend preschool.

Libertarianism (Egoism)

This position maintains a focus on the individual person and seeks a solution that is best for that person. The rights of each member of society are paramount. It is important to make certain that what the person wants is both legal and ethical.

Formalism (Deontological or Egalitarianism)

The focus of this theory is centered on the rules that govern a situation. Democratic principles are emphasized. Concepts of quality and comparable worth are paramount. Universality is the major theme guiding or directing the decision-making process.

An example of this theory is that every American citizen would be covered with basic health care insurance.

Deontology

Ethical principles guide a nurse's action, not the consequences of the actions. Deontology is Greek for duty. Ethical decisions are based on the duty of the nurse.

There are two types of deontology: act deontology and rule deontology.

Act Deontology

Actions are based on moral beliefs or values and result from the situation at hand. Actions are based on a duty to the patient.

Rule Deontology

Actions are based on rules and standards, which are fixed and inflexible. Actions are based on nursing standards of care and rules of law.

Humanitarianism (Fairness)

The focus of this theory is concerned with the distribution of benefits and burden in society. Concepts of fair opportunity, basic needs, and individual needs are emphasized. Fairness may not be the same as equality.

An example here is that every American would have a basic health insurance plan, but some individuals who could afford higher premiums could have a better health care plan than the basic plan.

Rawlsian Theory

This theory is from the philosopher John Rawls, who believed in social justice.

The focus of this theory is that one of the least advantaged should not be harmed. The overriding principle is justice. Each person is entitled to quality and access of medical care.

An example of this theory is that a fetus should not be harmed, as it cannot have its wishes known.

Naturalistic Theory

Focus of this theory is "it is what it ought to be." That is, if you have a terminal illness, you are meant to die. The major principle here is utmost rationality.

This theory also brings into the limelight the concept of futility. If treatment is futile, should such treatment interventions be funded?

Consequential Theory

The focus of this theory is scientism, that is, scientific and objective data guide the ethical decision-making process. No feelings enter into the equation. The basis is rationality and futility.

AN ETHICAL DECISION-MAKING MODEL

- Identify the problem.
- Tease out the ethical problem/dilemma.
- Gather objective and subjective data.
- Look at alternatives.
- Study the consequences of alternatives.
- Select the most appropriate alternative.
- Compare the selected alternative with the provider's own value/values system.

LANDMARK ETHICAL CASES

KAREN ANN QUINLAN

This was the first landmark case in the country. It happened in 1975 in the state of New Jersey. Karen Ann Quinlan had taken too many barbiturates and alcohol and subsequently landed in a persistent vegetative state. She was being maintained on a ventilator. The parents wanted her removed from the ventilator, as they stated that she would not want to live this way. The question was could a ventilator that was keeping one alive be removed. Was this ethical? This case made its way to the New Jersey State Supreme Court. The court made a decision in favor of the family. This court decision was based on the constitutional right of privacy in one's home. Such individuals can make decisions about patient care for ones that they love. It also permitted surrogate decision making, that is, when one is incompetent to make a decision, the surrogate can do so. The ventilator support was discontinued as a result of this court decision. Karen Ann Quinlan lived another 9 years off a ventilator. The court was also clear that they did not want to handle such cases. They recommended that every hospital in the state of New Jersey establish a bioethics committee to handle such ethical dilemmas because technology was now extending lives beyond expectations.

NANCY ELLEN JOBES

Nancy Ellen Jobes was involved in a motor vehicle accident. She was taken to a hospital in North Jersey, and her persistent vegetative state resulted from an anesthesia accident. She was tube fed for several years. She was married with 2 children, and her parents were still alive. Both the parents and her husband wanted the tube feeding discontinued. The question was could artificial food nutrition be discontinued. Is this a basic need for human life? This also was a New Jersey case, and the second case that went to the New Jersey State Supreme Court. The same attorney who represented the Quinlan case represented the Jobes case. The court decision was to allow artificial food and hydration to be discontinued. Nancy Ellen Jobes' tube feeding was discontinued, and she eventually died. The New Jersey State Supreme Court reinforced that such decisions should be made by health care providers and not courts.

NANCY BETH CRUZAN

This case is similar to that of Nancy Ellen Jobes. Nancy Beth Cruzan was involved in a motor vehicle accident. She was resuscitated at the scene, and she remained in a persistent vegetative state with tube feeding for several years. The parents decided that she would never want to live this way. Their attorney petitioned the Missouri State Supreme Court to hear their case. The court initially denied removal of the tube feeding, as they did not have clear and convincing evidence that Nancy Beth would not want to live this way. Cruzan's attorney petitioned the United States Supreme Court to hear the case, and the Court heard the case. If one was involved in ethics at the time, one was waiting for a decision from the United States Supreme Court regarding Nancy Beth Cruzan. The court did not hand down such a decision but stated that each state was like its own country and as such each state's court had to address such decisions. The Supreme Court clearly recommended that if patients had an advanced directive, then one's wishes could be known, thus providing clear evidence of how they would want to live. What resulted directly from the Cruzan case is the Patient Self-Determination Act of 1990. This act mandates that all health care facilities assess patients for an advanced directive on admission, and if they do not have an advanced directive but want one, the facility should assist the patient in securing an advanced directive. Many states have their own version of the Patient Self-Determination Act. What then happened to Nancy Beth Cruzan? The attorney for the Cruzans repetitioned the Missouri State Supreme Court to hear the case again. This time, individuals who knew Nancy Beth Cruzan testified as well as demonstrated through video how she was alive and active and would never want to live the rest of her life in a persistent vegetative state. The Supreme Court in Missouri this time made the decision to allow removal of the tube feeding. This was done, and Nancy Beth Cruzan died on December 26, 1990. One should take a look at Nancy Beth Cruzan's tombstone. On the top one can see a ventricular fibrillation pattern traced into the words "thank you." The tombstone reads Nancy Beth Cruzan, most loved daughter, sister, aunt. Born July 20, 1957. Departed January 11, 1983. At peace December 26, 1990. Her tombstone clearly illustrates the plight of a person who would want to die in peace without interventions that can sustain life but cannot provide quality of life.

TERRY SCHIAVO

Terri Schiavo had an eating disorder and most likely went into cardiac arrest from an electrolyte abnormality. She was resuscitated and lived several years in a hospice in Florida on tube feeding. The husband wanted the tube feeding discontinued, but the parents wanted the tube feeding to remain, as they felt that she was improving. This case went to the Florida State Supreme court. A nationally recognized neurologist also evaluated Terri Schiavo and determined that she was definitely in a persistent vegetative state. The Florida State Supreme Court ruled that the tube feeding could be removed. The parents were very upset with this decision and requested their attorney to petition the United States Supreme Court to hear the case. The United States Supreme Court refused to hear the case, making the Florida State Supreme Court decision final. The tube feeding was discontinued and Terri Schiavo died. What is interesting in this case and is very typical of ethical dilemmas is the discordance among the family. The reality is that the husband had the right to make the decision. The Florida State Supreme Court thus ruled.

There are many ethical encounters today. Some examples are advanced directives and the right to live or die, active or passive euthanasia, do-not-resuscitate orders, the rights of the dying client, use of life-saving equipment, human cloning, research on mentally impaired patients, research on embryos, organ donation issues, operative issues, and incompetent health care providers.

Common causes of ethical dilemmas are guilt of a family member; lack of agreement among family members; poor communication, such as a lack of information or incorrect communication; and conflicting core values.

CASE VIGNETTE

This is the case of Mr. J, a 79-year-old Caucasian male. He had a massive cerebrovascular accident on his right side with the resultant left-sided paralysis. The patient was on a ventilator and sedated. The wife requested that the ventilation be discontinued. The physician consulted the ethics committee to review the case. The committee at this particular hospital was advisory in nature. Three members of the committee reviewed this case. They spoke to the physician and reviewed the patient's medical record. In the record was a clearly executed advance directive. They then went and assessed the patient. One of the committee members was a nurse who was a clinical specialist in neurology. The patient was not moving and maintained on a ventilator. This nurse through a series of questions with the patient raising his index finger for yes and his middle finger for no clearly demonstrated that the patient could understand what was being said. The patient through this type of communication clearly indicated that he wanted to live and did not want to be removed from the ventilator. The ethics committee discussed this case, and their recommendation was to leave the patient on the ventilator. This was discussed with both the physician as well as the patient's wife. The patient's wife was at first distraught with this information. But after the committee members demonstrated to her how the patient could clearly hear them and make his wishes known, the wife agreed that the patient should remain on the ventilator. The patient died 10 days later on the ventilator. This case clearly indicates that hearing is the last sense to go and that part of ethics case consultation is talking to the patient even if he or she seems to be totally neurologically obtunded. It is an excellent case of patient autonomy and one that shows that patients can be mentally sound even if sedated on a ventilator.

More and more states are passing assisted suicide legislation. Five states have done so as of the writing of this book. Thus far the client must commit the act themselves, for example, a caregiver could put a large amount of pills in front of the client, but the caregiver could not help the client take the medication.

BUSINESS ETHICS

The reality is that health care organizations are businesses. As such one must comply with business ethics and principles.

Billing practices must be legal and ethical and follow federal and state guidelines. There are pressures on administrators today to balance cost with quality. There is usually always room for operational efficiency and cost containment; however, patient care and nursing care must suffer at the expense of too aggressive cost-cutting measures. Such measures also create ethical dilemmas for nurse executives. One has to recognize that such conflicts will exist, and it is recommended that nurse executives develop a plan to handle such dilemmas. There is a fine balance between corporate demands for cost containment and bottom line performance versus proper staffing and quality patient care.

LEGAL ISSUES

This section discusses legal issues. An overview of law and legal terminology, nursing negligence and contributing factors, practice settings and legal issues, and the major elements of malpractice is discussed.

The reality is that health care is a very dynamic practice environment. There is an increasing awareness on the part of the public about quality care as well as malpractice litigation. As nurses we have the duty to provide care. We do not want to breach that care. We want to provide safe practice, and we want to be vigilant in preventing liability.

The reason why law exists is that when 2 parties cannot mutually resolve an issue they can have it adjudicated by the legal system.

There are different types of law:

- Public versus private
- Criminal versus noncriminal
- Case versus code based

Public law is constitutional law. It includes both administrative law and criminal law and defines a citizen to government relationship. Private law is civil law. This defines citizen to citizen relationships and includes personal responsibilities about things we own, injuries we inflict, and contracts that we make or break.

Criminal law involves the federal or state government. It is where one prosecutes an offense against society or attempts to deprive personal liberty or life. And the legal system requires proof beyond reasonable doubt.

Noncriminal or civil law involves disputes between 2 parties, which is often settled with an exchange of money. In a court it requires convincing a jury that the complaint is true.

Case law is known as common law. When one thinks about it, the English initially settled in the United States in colonies. Thus, in most of our states, we have adopted the English system of law known as case law or common law. Case law or common law is created by judges and is nonstatutory in nature. The premise is that when a decision is made by a court, that decision sets precedents for future cases that are similar.

Code law was created by Napoleon Bonaparte in France. It is a collection of laws created by legislation. In essence, a governmental body tries to address every act of human behavior through a statute or law. Thus, if you violate the law, you are guilty. The one state in the United States that is predominantly code based is the state of Louisiana, as Louisiana was settled by French colonists from Nova Scotia.

A good example of statutory law is local governments passing laws that have an influence on the lives of individuals. Known as ordinances these local laws are also subject to review by the courts. One example is public health. Some states refer to this as police power. By this they do not mean the power of the police department but the power of public health. There are statutes, for example, whereby a public health organization can quarantine individuals with a communicable disease. This example authorizes the establishment of a Board of Health to administer legislative mandates, such as prevention of human communicable diseases and regulation of health care facilities.

To understand law one must understand the Latin language. The following are key concepts that define the legal system in the United States.

- Res Judicata
- Stare Decisis
- Respondeat Superior
- Charitable Immunity
- Res Ipsa Loquitur

Res Judicata

Res Judicata implies that the thing has been decided. In other words, at some point there is a final decision or judgment and the 2 parties cannot petition the courts again for the same issue.

Stare Decisis

Stare Decisis implies to stand by that which has been decided. This relates to the final decision that sets precedent that should not afterward be deviated from. The only thing that changes this concept is when technology changes or there is a major societal shift. A great example here is what has been discussed previously about the Karen Ann Quinlan case where technology was keeping her alive, even though she was in a persistent vegetative state. Normally the court would have ruled not to discontinue the ventilator support, but secondary to the change in technology the New Jersey state Supreme Court decided otherwise.

Respondeat Superior

Respondeat Superior implies let the master speak. This relates to our role as nurse executives and includes concepts of vicarious liability, the borrowed servant doctrine, and captain of the ship rule. Vicarious liability implies that one can be liable as a manager for what his or her subordinate or employee does. This can be applicable only if the manager has knowledge that the employee is doing something wrong and takes no action. An example is an employee who makes multiple medication errors, the manager knows this, but does not address it. Should a major error occur that harms the patient, both the employee and the manager can be held accountable. The borrowed servant doctrine relates to borrowing an employee from another entity. An example in nursing is the use of agency nurses. They are employed by an agency, yet the hospital uses their services. They are then a borrowed servant for the hospital, and the hospital can be held accountable if the nurses are not competent to do what they are supposed to do; thus both entities, the agency and the hospital, could be sued if a procedure is done incorrectly.

Medical staff have been sued under this doctrine (Showalter & Southwick, 1999). It involves the concept of peer review. Even though one may be an independent practitioner contracted to provide services, the medical staff could be sued if a physician is not competent to perform certain procedures and they perform them and a medical error results.

Charitable Immunity

Should one go back into the history of hospitals, they initially were charitable organizations. They were nonprofit organizations. Thus they were immune from lawsuits, as how could one sue an organization that is providing free care. Over time hospitals have become businesses, and as such they can be sued like any other business. Immunity is never absolute. Negligent conduct can nullify any charitable immunity doctrine. Examples are willful, wanton, gross, or reckless behaviors. Most states have abandoned their charitable immunity doctrines. Some states have a dollar amount that the organization would pay out if sued.

Res Ipsa Loquitur

Res Ipsa Loquitur implies the action speaks for itself. Cases that fall under this concept are not defensible in court. An example is a retained lap sponge after a surgical procedure. The preoperative X-ray demonstrates no lap sponge, whereas the postoperative X-ray demonstrates one. This would be indefensible in court, as clearly there is evidence that documents that the sponge count was incorrect in the operating room. These cases should be settled out of court by the organization offering to settle.

Tort

A tort is a civil wrong other than a breach of contract. The law addresses negligence and professional negligence and protects others from unreasonable and foreseeable risk of harm. The law provides a remedy for the injured person to seek damages. Negligence is conduct that falls below the standard established by law or by our accrediting bodies or licensing boards. It is protection from unreasonable risk of harm and includes the concept of foreseeability. In other words, if I could foresee that I was negligent in some manner and that the patient would suffer from this negligence, then most likely there could be a potential lawsuit.

Professional negligence or professional malpractice is the conduct of professionals that falls below the professional standard of due care. It is conduct of care that falls below the standard minimum of specialized knowledge and ability. It is important to understand that standards of care can be both national and regional.

There also is liability for health care systems and the breach of duty owed to its patients. It is implied that health care facilities will maintain a safe environment with safe state-of-the-art equipment; that the health care facility will provide competent, qualified, and trained licensed individuals to provide care; that the facility will provide proper orientation and supervision of staff; and that the facility will maintain appropriate policies, procedures, and bylaws.

So how then does one get sued? Let us review the anatomy of a malpractice case. There are 5 key elements.

1. The duty to provide care
2. A breach in the duty to provide care
3. A tort is committed (usually an act of negligence)
4. An untoward outcome results
5. The events were foreseeable

First there is the duty to provide care. One way health care providers can get into trouble is if they do not provide the care when they should. For example, a patient suffers cardiac arrest and no one does cardiopulmonary resuscitation. Another way that health care providers can be sued is if a negligent act is committed. It is crucial to understand that negligent acts can be acts that we commit and just as important omit. Whether we breach the duty to provide care or commit a negligent act, there must be an untoward outcome that results. In other words, one can commit a negligent act but no harm comes to the patient; then there really is no reason for the patient to sue; however, some patients complain about mental anguish as some vague negative outcome. One of the key concepts is that the events were foreseeable. For example: a patient has an intravenous catheter that infiltrates. The nurse applies a warm compress. The compress is made by running a wash rag under hot water, placing it in a blue chux pad, and microwaving the chux pad. This then is applied to the site of infiltration, and the patient suffers a second-degree burn. The nurse did not follow the procedure for applying a warm compress safely, which is through a controlled method of heating not microwaving. Should the patient sue, the nurse would most likely be liable, as the nurse committed an act of negligence, and it is forseeable that when you heat something in a microwave oven the inside temperature could be extreme that could burn a patient.

The way to prevent malpractice is to make certain that individuals follow the standards of care, do not take shortcuts, and continually assess patient's status. Documentation is also critical. What are some professional negligence claims against nurses? These are based almost exclusively on personal injury that results from various types of negligent conduct and could also involve product liability and most recently complementary and alternative health care options. Other potential liabilities include failure to provide for patient safety; failure to properly assess and diagnose a patient; incorrectly treating a patient, for example, providing the wrong medication; failure to collaborate with the physician when necessary; and failure to look for other causes of illness when the patient is not responding to treatment. Some common allegations of negligent conduct are an inadequate assessment, inadequate communication, poor documentation, improper use of equipment, and failure to follow policy, procedure, and protocol.

Contract Law

Contract law includes promises that have been made. It is enforced once a legal right is created. In nursing it can involve the nurse employer, nurse manager, nurse practitioner, or nurse entrepreneur. A contract is a voluntary agreement for the benefit of 2 or more individuals that is legally qualified. Some states include verbal contracts as well.

Consents

Consents can be verbal, written, applied, and informed. An example of a verbal consent is when a patient permits to have the blood work drawn. An example of written consent is an operative permit. Implied consent occurs when the patient cannot sign or give verbal consent, for example, when a patient codes it is implied that we should resuscitate him or her. Another example of implied consent is that once the patient signs a consent form for admission and treatment, it is implied that you will have laboratory work done, X-rays, diagnostics, etc.

Other Legal Issues

Sexual harassment is a legal issue. Sexual harassment is not just sexual favors for job advancement. It can be unwanted sexual remarks made in the workplace. Another legal issue is violation of the Fair Labor Standards Act, which covers age discrimination. Employees older than 40 years are protected. Most employees in most settings are employees at will. This protects both the employer and the employee. Employment can be ended at the will of either party for good reason, bad reason, or no reason. This is how health care organizations can do layoffs when they need to downsize.

Defenses against allegations of professional negligence include untimely filing of the case, for example, the plaintiff files a case after the statute of limitations runs out. In most states the statute of limitation for adults is 2 years from discovery of a problem. Another defense is known as the assumption of risk: the patient knew it was dangerous, had the facts about the danger, and chose to take on the danger. An example is an experimental drug that the patient consents to take. Another defense is immunity from suit. An example is the Good Samaritan Act. This act covers laypeople who respond to help others in time of need, for example, a motor vehicle accident. One should not be sued if he or she acts in good faith to help another who is in danger; however, when a health care provider responds, one is held to a higher standard, that is, he or she better do what a qualified health provider would do and better not abandon the patient.

The best defense is a good offense. Harm to a patient can arise from intentional or unintentional acts. Intentional acts of harm can include defamation, invasion of privacy, assault and battery, imprisonment, or infliction of emotional distress. Unintentional acts of harm can include omission or negligence.

References

American Nurses Association. (2015). *Code of ethics with interpretative statements.* Silver Spring, MD: American Nurses Association.

Guido, G. W. (2013). *Legal & ethical issues in nursing* (6th ed.). New York City, NY: Pearson Education.

Showalter, J. S., & Southwick, A. F. (1999). *Southwick's the law of health care administration* (3rd ed.). Chicago, IL: Health Administration Press/American College of Health Care Executives.

CHAPTER

9

Budgeting and Financial Management

Al Rundio

This chapter will review:

HEALTH CARE REIMBURSEMENT IN THE UNITED STATES

FINANCIAL TERMS

OPERATING BUDGET

CAPITAL BUDGET

SAMPLE BUDGET

BUDGET REPORTS

This chapter covers budgeting and financial management for nurse executives. The topics that we will cover are the following:

- What is budgeting
- Benefits of budgeting
- How is it used
- Types of budgets
- Operating versus capital budgets

Whether an organization is for-profit or not-for-profit, the goal is to turn a positive bottom-line whereby revenues exceed expenses. This is where revenue comes from:

- Medicare
- Medicaid
- Managed care organizations
- Fee-for-service
- Diagnostic-related groups (DRGs)
- Private insurers

- Health maintenance organizations (HMOs)
- Preferred provider organizations (PPOs)
- Independent professional associations (IPAs)
- Capitation
- Accountable care organizations (ACOs)
- Self-pay patients
- Contributions

Medicare consists of 4 parts.

Medicare Part A covers 100% of inpatient care for the first 20 days in a nursing home; after that it will cover 80% of the cost for the next 80 days.

Medicare Part B covers outpatient care, such as primary care, durable medical equipment, physical therapy, and other like services.

Medicare Part C plans are referred to as the Medicare advantage plans. Other insurance companies manage patients who have Medicare.

Medicare Part D was created under the Medicare Modernization Act of 2003 signed into law by President George W. Bush. One of the key components of this Act was the creation of Medicare Part D and the prescription drug plan. The prescription drug plan covers a set amount per year, and then patients fall into what is known as the doughnut hole whereby they have to pay cash for their prescriptions for the rest of the year, and then in the new year the prescription plan will cover again the same set amount as previously.

Managed care organizations consist of a variety of insurance products where the insurance company manages costs, for example, a patient who is hyperthyroid may need to get a baseline ultrasound imaging done before the insurance company authorizes a nuclear scan of the thyroid gland.

Fee-for-service is when a provider or a hospital charges a set fee to the insurance company per visit or per hospital day. Insurance companies are trying to move away from a fee-for-service provider scale.

DRG stands for diagnostic-related group. This form of reimbursement was implemented in 1981 in pilot states. The idea of the DRG system is to reimburse on a case basis rather than on a fee-for-service basis. For example, reimbursement in a hospital would occur for a case rather than as daily charges. The key to reimbursement under the DRG system was the medical coder in the medical records department. This was a system of averages in which case rates were established based on the average length of stay. It is important to recognize that this system was adopted nationally by the Medicare system, and under Medicare Part A for inpatient hospital care, reimbursement occurs through the DRG system.

The DRG system created a system of peer review for physicians. It created a new role for nursing, that of the Utilization Review Coordinator (URC). It also created a new role for the medical staff. For a hospital to bill its own services under DRG, it had to have a Utilization Review Committee of the Medical Staff and a Utilization Review Department in the hospital. Members of the medical staff on this committee serve as physician advisors to the URC. Admissions and length of stay had to be justified. Within 24 hours of admission the medical record had to be reviewed by the URC. The URC had to be a registered nurse. This nurse had to look for 2 major components on the medical record: severity of illness and intensity of service. In other words, the patient had to have a valid diagnosis for admission as well as a service that could be provided only by a hospital inpatient service. The URC also reviewed the medical record periodically for continued length of stay. Admissions could be denied, continued length of stay could be denied, or a change in level of care could result, for example, a change to a nursing home rate of payment if the patient was just awaiting nursing home placement. There could also be carve-out days when the URC would carve out set days when acute services were not rendered. In case of an admission denial, a continued stay denial, a change in the level of care, or carve-out days, the medical record had to be referred by the URC to the physician advisor from the medical staff. The physician advisor would review the medical record and speak with the patient's attending physician. The physician advisor would either agree with the URC referral or could approve further continued stay. Often more documentation by the attending physician was just needed to justify the admission or continued stay. The insurance company would then not be responsible for payment of carve-out days or continued stay if either the admission or continued stay was denied. Whenever a decision such as admission denial or continued length of stay denial was made, the patient would be provided with a letter advising him or her that he or she had 24 hours after which time the insurance company would no longer pay. There were 3 levels for appeal by the patient. A state-appointed peer review organization oversaw and monitored the system in each hospital.

Utilization review was the precursor to case management as we know it today.

Private insurance companies exist to cover health care expenditures. Today usually they follow a managed care model.

HMO is a health maintenance organization. These organizations came about in the 1970s. Their focus was on preventative services. Often HMOs would have their own clinics and even hospitals or would contract with hospitals to manage patient care.

PPO is a preferred provider organization. These organizations contract with set providers and hospitals and other types of service providers to manage the cost of patient care.

IPA is an independent professional association or an independent physician association. A group of providers establish an insurance plan and manage patient care and costs within that set group of providers.

Capitation came about in the late 1990s. Capitation is gaining momentum in the vast variety of insurance products in the market. In capitation, payments are made per member per month regardless of whether the services are accessed or not and regardless of the number of times a patient accesses his or her service in a given month. For example, primary care providers may be reimbursed $10 per month for each patient enrolled in the capitated model. They will receive this dollar amount regardless of the care provided. The goal for providers is to keep the patient out of the practice, as they are paid whether the patient is seen in the practice or not. The focus for the provider then becomes using certain preventative strategies to keep the patient healthy. Hospitals and other health services can also be part of a capitated model whereby they are also paid a monthly fee per member per month.

Self-pay patients are patients who do not have insurance and pay for care themselves.

Contributions can be used for patient care. Usually this comes from philanthropy or other activities that an organization uses to raise money.

Value-based purchasing has become important. What value is the patient receiving by purchasing certain organizations' health care services? For example, one hospital system has one guaranteed price regardless of the outcome. For example, if a patient has a surgical procedure done and then develops a wound infection postoperatively requiring readmission, neither the patient nor the insurance company is charged for the additional hospital stay. The focus of value-based purchasing is to provide quality care to patients in a cost-effective manner.

ACOs were a key component of the Patient Protection and Affordable Care Act signed into law by President Barack Obama in 2010. The U.S. health care delivery system has been billing in silos, that is, each service bills independently of the other. The new model of care delivery is that of an ACO. This is where the services send one bundled bill and then share the reimbursement received. The key to maximizing reimbursement in an ACO is to have good quality care, as the reimbursement then tends to be higher. If the organization is accountable, then the services police each other so that quality care occurs in all services. One of the key aspects of an ACO is that of the medical home, which can be primary care or a clinic that oversees the patient's care throughout the system.

Another important aspect of maximizing revenue in a hospital is that of the Hospital Consumer Assessment of Health Provider Survey. This survey evaluates the patient experience. The patient experience ties to hospital value-based purchasing domains. In Medicare 70% reimbursement was based on the process of care and 30% was based on the patient experience. The process of care defines certain criteria that must be met per diagnosis. For example, if a patient has chest pain, certain procedures must be done, such as cardiac enzymes, troponin levels, electrocardiography, portable chest X-ray, and other clinical care factors. If the criteria are not met, then for that particular case they would receive a lower score below 70%. The same occurs with the patient experience; if certain satisfaction scores are not met, then the case will receive less than 30% for the patient experience. These dollar amounts would then be subtracted from the DRG case rate. The new value-based purchasing domains center on 4 aspects of care: the clinical process of care, patient experience, efficiency, and quality.

Businesses are concerned with 3 major concepts:

- Assets
- Liabilities
- Equity

ASSETS

Resources owned

Stated as current assets-fixed assets and noncurrent assets

Current assets are cash and other assets that can be turned into cash within 1 year

LIABLITIES

Opposite of assets

Obligations to be paid

Current liabilities are obligations that are due within the year, e.g., wages, accounts, taxes

Long-term liabilities are obligations or debts that are not due within 1 year, e.g., mortgage, loans

EQUITY

Associated with assets and liabilities
Excess of assets over liabilities
Resources invested by the owner
May be called fund balance or net worth
A charge master is maintained by accounting for all expenses and revenues

Development of the Annual Budget

The budget process is ongoing and dynamic. It provides feedback. The budget process includes collecting data, analyzing the data, planning activities and services, developing and implementing a plan, and evaluating the outcomes. The following chart indicates what types of data are collected and the sources from where data are extrapolated.

Types of Data	Sources of Data
Payer mix	Statistical reports
Patient mix	Historical information
Patient acuity	Organizational goals and objectives
Case mix index	Industry trends in the marketplace
Staff mix	
Standards of care	
Patient outcomes	
Hours of care per patient-day	
Plan for change in services/resources	

In developing a budget a manager has to forecast the resources required to deliver the anticipated services. He or she needs to set goals, design the budget, submit it for approval, and defend it.

Part of monitoring the budget is to evaluate outcomes whereby actual revenues and costs are compared with projected revenues and costs. It is important to identify variances by analyzing cost, efficiency, and volume variances. Based on this analysis goals may need to be modified, a change in the level or type of service may be required, and a change in the level of resources used may be required. The most common type of variance is generally caused by cost and efficiency. This would involve paying too much for the care delivered, for example, use of agency nurses and also providing more than projected hours of nursing care.

Comprehensive data collection is involved in developing the budget. When the forecast is based on such data collection, the actual outcomes should come close to the predicted outcomes.

The 2 major types of budgets are the operating and the capital budget.

An operating budget represents a financial quantification of the organization's goals and objectives and, most importantly, how those goals and objectives are going to be achieved. This budget is one of management's most widely used tools. The key is to receive timely reports and, most importantly, take action on any variances in those reports.

The budget should be the result of a joint effort by the administration and management team as to what exactly the organization's operating plans are for the future.

There are different types of budgets. Zero-based budgeting is ideal for new services, a major paradigm shift or change in the health care delivery system, especially how care is reimbursed, and it is also used as a check and balance on the organization's budget. The zero-based budget is a tabula rasa (blank slate) where one justifies each revenue and expense item.

Most organizations embrace historical budgeting. This is where prior actual budget experience, usually for a 3- to 5-year period, is used to project the next fiscal budget.

It is important to know the organization's budget cycle. There are 3 budget cycles:

January 1 to December 31
July 1 to June 30
October 1 to September 30

It is important to note that the Centers for Medicare and Medicaid Services is on an October 1 to September 30 budget cycle.

When developing the budget, it is important to view the current and the projected reimbursement systems, for example, going from a fee-for-service system to a capitated system. It is also important to estimate any inflation factors, such as fringe benefits, supplies, pharmaceuticals, food, energy, and staff salaries.

The operational budget includes the FTEs, that is, the full-time equivalents. The national definition is that an FTE is equal to 2080 paid hours, which includes benefit time. Included in the 2080 hours are both productive time and nonproductive time. Each organization defines its own nonproductive time, which is paid time off. More than one employee can make up 1.0 FTE, for example, 2 employees may each work 20 hours or 0.5 FTE; thus 2 employees would equal 1.0 FTE. The formula for calculating FTEs includes budgeted patient-days, budgeted nursing hours per patient-day, budgeted staff hours, and budgeted nonproductive time.

BUDGET EXAMPLE

You are a nursing executive. You have the following data available to you:

A total of 5.0 hours of nursing care per patient-day.

An average daily census of 30 patients per day.

Staff receive the following benefits: 30 days paid time off per year.

How many FTEs do you need to staff the unit?

First take the 30 patients per day × 365 days per year = 10,950 patient-days for the year.

Next take the 10,950 patient-days × 5.0 staffed hours = 54,750 total staffed hours for the year.

Now take the 54,750 staffed hours divided by 2080 hours (what one FTE works).

54,750 divided by 2080 = 26.32. You will need 26.32 FTEs to staff the unit to deliver 5 hours of care per patient-day. The problem is that those 2080 hours are inclusive of hours for paid time off. Because the question advised that each employee gets 30 days of benefit time, subtract the benefit days in hours from the 2080 hours. Regardless of what shift an employee works, most organizations consider a benefit day to equal 8 hours of pay. Therefore, 30 × 8 = 240 hours of paid time off.

Subtract the 240 hours from the 2080 total hours: 2080–240 = 1840 productive hours.

Now divide the 54,750 staffed hours by 1840 productive hours to get the real FTEs needed to staff the unit.

54,750 divided by 1840 = 29.75 FTEs.

The reasons for including the paid time off in the formulas is that, if you divide by 2080 hours, the unit will either be short staffed when staff take vacation time or you will have to deliver the hours of care by paying overtime or bonus dollars or hiring agency staff, which is costly.

Productive time generally includes actual hours worked and overtime hours worked. Some organizations count meeting time, educational time, and orientation time as productive hours; others do not.

Nonproductive time includes vacation time, holiday time, and bereavement time. Some organizations consider meeting time, educational time, and orientation time as nonproductive hours; some organizations consider these hours as productive hours.

Capital Budget

The capital budget includes items to be purchased that will last for more than a year. They are defined as capital acquisitions. There are 2 major types of capital budgets, that of major movable equipment and that of fixed assets. An example of fixed assets is renovation of the classroom that would remain in place for years to come. Most nurse executives deal with the major movable equipment budget. To prepare a major movable equipment budget properly, one needs to know what minimum dollar amount the organization has established as to what gets budgeted in the major movable capital equipment budget. This dollar amount varies by organization. Generally, this dollar amount is anywhere from $500 to $5000. In addition to knowing the dollar amount, one also needs to know the depreciation value of the piece of equipment, that is, what is the expected life of the piece of equipment. The rationale for this is that, to maintain state-of-the-art equipment, one has to plan for future capital expense as the equipment depreciates.

Capital budgets are large outlays of money that require special attention. Some examples of capital budget items are cardiac monitors, computers, computed tomography scanners, and magnetic resonance imaging scanners.

Budget Reports

To manage a budget well, it is important for nurse executives to have timely reports that they can understand. Data from some reports may include the number of beds in service by unit, the number of admissions, the patient-days, length of stay, average daily census, percentage occupancy rate, FTEs staffed, hours staffed, and hours per patient-day. Regarding staffing data reports, some report the hours worked by registered nurses, licensed practical nurses, patient care technicians, supervisors and department heads, technicians, clerical workers, and other professionals. Most of these reports run at the time that payroll is completed, that is, if an organization is paid every 2 weeks, these reports run every 2 weeks. It is critical that nurse executives review the reports, identify variances, and most importantly take corrective action.

For further information on finance and budgeting for nurse managers please refer to Rundio (2016a).

Resources

Rundio, A. (2012). *Budgeting & finance for nurse managers.* Indianapolis, IN: Sigma Theta Tau International.

Rundio, A. (2016a). *The nurse manager's guide to budgeting & finance* (2nd ed.). Indianapolis, IN: Sigma Theta Tau Publications.

Rundio, A. (2016b). *Budgeting & finance for nurse managers* (2nd ed.). Indianapolis, IN: Sigma Theta Tau International.

Rundio, A., Wilson, V., & Meloy, F. (2016c). *The nurse executive review and resource manual* (3rd ed.). Silver Spring, MD: ANA Publications.

CHAPTER

10

Health Policy

Al Rundio

This chapter will review:

THE 5 TYPES OF HEALTH POLICY

THE COMPOSITION OF THE HEALTH CARE WORKFORCE IN THE UNITED STATES

POLITICS

PROCESS OF HOW A BILL BECOMES A LAW

There are 5 types of health policy:

1. Public policy involves government bodies.
2. Social policy promotes public welfare and addresses health disparities such as reimbursement of care and/or access to care.
3. Health policy involves decisions made to promote the health of individual citizens.
4. Institutional policy governs the workplace.
5. Organizational policies are positions taken by organizations.

See a snapshot of the U.S. workforce on the next page.

Trend of Employment Statistics for Healthcare Practitioners and Technical Occupations (2013 - 2017)

Occupation	2013		2014		2015		2016		2017		5-Year Growth/Loss
	Employed	% of Field	Employed	% of Field	Employed	% of Field	Employed	% of Field	Employed	% of Field	
Chiropractors	28,850	0.4%	29,830	0.4%	32,080	0.4%	32,960	0.4%	33,630	0.4%	17%
Dentists	112,300	1.4%	115,390	1.5%	116,750	1.5%	122,330	1.5%	125,300	1.5%	12%
Dietitians and Nutritionists	59,530	0.8%	59,490	0.8%	59,740	0.7%	61,430	0.7%	62,980	0.7%	6%
EMTs and Paramedics	237,660	3.1%	235,760	3.0%	236,890	3.0%	244,960	2.9%	251,860	3.0%	6%
Health Diagnosing and Treating Practitioners (Audiologists, Podiatrists, etc.)	689,450	8.9%	704,140	9.0%	723,530	9.0%	748,880	9.0%	773,280	9.1%	12%
LPNS and LVNs	705,200	9.1%	695,610	8.9%	697,250	8.7%	702,400	8.4%	702,700	8.3%	0%
Nursing (Registered and Advanced Practice)	**2,816,150**	**36.3%**	**2,851,060**	**36.3%**	**2,928,810**	**36.5%**	**3,053,540**	**36.7%**	**3,122,270**	**36.7%**	**11%**
Optometrists	32,040	0.4%	33,340	0.4%	35,300	0.4%	36,430	0.4%	37,240	0.4%	16%
Pharmacists	287,420	3.7%	290,780	3.7%	295,620	3.7%	305,510	3.7%	309,330	3.6%	8%
Physician Assistants	88,110	1.1%	91,670	1.2%	98,470	1.2%	104,050	1.3%	109,220	1.3%	24%
Physicians and Surgeons	623,380	8.0%	633,480	8.1%	642,720	8.0%	649,850	7.8%	666,490	7.8%	7%
Technicians and Technologists	2,016,520	26.0%	2,051,370	26.1%	2,088,980	26.0%	2,188,520	26.3%	2,243,070	26.4%	11%
Veterinarians	59,230	0.8%	62,470	0.8%	65,650	0.8%	67,650	0.8%	69,370	0.8%	17%

The Total Employment by Occupation comparing May 2013 with May 2017

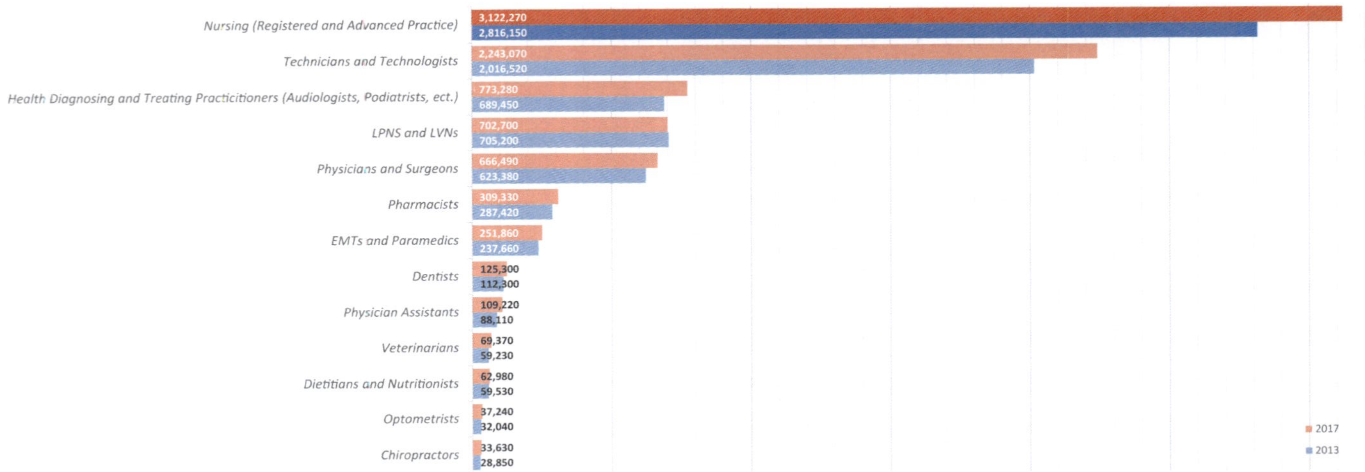

Bureau of Labor Statistics. Occupational Employment Statistics, 2013-2017. Public-use file. https://www.bls.gov/oes/tables.htm

EMT, emergency medical technicians; LPN, licensed practical nurse; LVN, licensed vocational nurse.

Nursing is the largest workforce in health care, far exceeding other professionals; therefore, nurses are in a pivotal position to have a major impact on health policy.

Health policy is a complex and multidimensional dynamic process (Huber, 2013). It reflects the values of those setting the agenda. Conflict can result when policies affect private issues, such as smoking.

There is an increased focus on the following:

- Quality of health care through prevention and consumer health literacy
- Accessibility to health care
- Financial strength and sustainability of Medicare and other programs
- Care of the elderly and initiatives to improve the quality of life of these patients
- Nursing's involvement in the political process to affect the health of patients, families, communities, and populations (Mason et al., 2016)

How can nursing get involved in health policy?

Here are some ways in which nurses can engage in health policy:

- Grassroots efforts such as writing or sending email to your congressional representatives and their aides
- Connecting with congressional representatives to sponsor key legislation affecting nursing practice and the nation's health
- Political advocacy
- Running for a political office, such as a Freeholder, Mayor of a town, Public Health Officer, Commissioner or Assistant Commissioner of Health, Senator, Congressional Representative, Governor

The following section describes how a bill becomes a law.

A senator or congressional representative introduces a bill. He/she sends it to the clerk of the respective house (either the senate or the House of Representatives). The clerk gives the bill a number and title. This is considered the first reading. The bill is then referred to a proper committee of the house where it is sponsored, for example, the Senate Finance and Budget Committee. This committee may decide that the bill is not necessary and table it, which kills the bill at once. It would have to be responsored at a future date. The committee may decide that the bill is worthwhile and hold hearings to listen to facts and opinion presented by experts and other interested persons. After members of the committee have debated the bill and perhaps offered amendments, a vote is taken, and if the vote is favorable, the bill is sent back to the floor of the house for a vote. The clerk reads the bill sentence by sentence to the house; this is known as the second reading. Members are then permitted to debate the bill and offer amendments. In the House of Representatives the time for debate is limited by what is termed a cloture rule, but there is no such restriction in the Senate, where 60 votes are required. This can create a filibuster where one or more opponents hold the floor to defeat the bill. The third reading is by title only, and the bill is then put to a vote. Vote can occur by voice or roll call. Members who are not present for the vote but who wish to record their vote may be paired if each negative vote has a balancing affirmative one. Should the bill pass the first house, it is then sent to the other house of Congress where it may be defeated or passed with or without amendments. If the bill is defeated it dies. Should amendments be made to the bill, then a joint congressional committee must be appointed by both houses to iron out the differences. The bill is then sent back to the house of origin for a vote; if passed, it is then sent to the other house for a vote. After final passage by both houses the bill is sent to the President. The President can sign the bill, and then it becomes law, or can veto the bill by not signing the bill and send it back to the house of origin stating the reasons for the veto. The objections of the bill would be read by the house of origin and debated. A roll call vote is then taken. The bill must receive a two-thirds or greater vote for the bill to be sent to the other house of Congress. The other house must also approve the bill by a two-thirds or greater vote. If both houses approve the bill by a two-thirds or greater vote, the President's veto is overridden and the bill becomes law. If either house does not vote favorably by two-thirds or more, the bill is defeated and goes no further. The President's veto is then upheld. There are 2 other interesting processes that can happen. Should the President decide not to sign or veto the bill, he or she may retain it for 10 days (Sundays do not count). Following the 10 days the bill would automatically become law without signature. One can question why the President would do this. The President's party may not want the bill but the President may. So, for political reasons he or she may elect not to sign the bill but allow it to become law without his or her signature. What is far more interesting is that should Congress adjourn within those 10 days, the bill is automatically killed. This process of indirect rejection is known as a pocket veto. So, if the President wants to veto the bill, it is actually safer for him or her not to sign the bill if Congress is adjourning within that 10-day period.

References

Huber, D. (2013). *Leadership and nursing care management* (5th ed.). Philadelphia: Saunders/Elsevier.

Mason, D. J., Gardner, D. B., Outlaw, F. H., & O'Grady, E. T. (Eds.). (2016). *Policy & politics in nursing & health care* (7th ed.). St. Louis, MO: Elsevier.

CHAPTER

11

Career Planning

William J. Lorman

This chapter will review:

PLANNING BY THE INDIVIDUAL

TERMS RELATED TO CAREER

DEVELOPING SHORT-TERM, INTERMEDIATE, AND LONG-TERM GOALS IN THE CAREER PLANNING PROCESS

MODELS USED IN PLANNING

THE PROCESS OF CAREER PLANNING

PLANNING BY HEALTH CARE ORGANIZATIONS

SUCCESSION PLANNING

USING A CAREER COUNSELOR

USING A MENTOR

Because of the impending retirement of large numbers of people from the baby boomer era, there is expected to be a gap of skilled workers available to fill positions in the health care industry. In addition, the health care industry is further adversely affected by the growth trends because of demographic shifts and a decrease in the overall health of the U.S. population. Baby boomers themselves are the largest demographic group in the country, with a population of around 76 million, and this population will require the use of health care services more frequently (Randstad North America, 2000). These trends are forcing health care organizations to strategically plan for growth through expansion of both facilities and workforce. Health care organizations are called upon to develop employees and managers to fill vacancies created by all these trends mentioned. Career development programs can provide health care organizations with one solution to close the experience and supply gap as they prepare for this turbulent future. These programs assess the needs of the organization and its employees and devise a strategic plan to fill future needs through retention of key workers and by developing the employees to fill future needs.

PLANNING BY THE INDIVIDUAL

Career planning is one of the most important aspects for professionals, especially those pursuing a career in the health care industry. It is a function that should be appraised on a continuous basis by the student, applicant, candidate, and even those already in a job where a promotion, change, or new challenge is sought after. Although most people have expectations about their career, the main expectation is finding a position related to their educational and/or experiential field.

TERMS RELATED TO CAREER

According to dictionary.reference.com, career is defined as an occupation or profession, especially one requiring special training and followed as one's lifework. Sometimes, a person can move into different careers based on a number of factors such as a person's ongoing education, newly identified openings in a specific area, or lack of demand for a current career path. The following are other terms related to "career":

- Career planning is the process by which one selects career goals and the career path to accomplish those goals (Werther & Davis, 1993). To start the process of career planning, a list of personal abilities and desires of the individual should be developed along with any experience already accomplished.
- Career management is the combination of structured planning and the active management choice of one's own professional career.
- Career orientation refers to the overall design or pattern of one's career, shaped by particular goals and interests and identifiable by particular positions that embody these goals and interests.
- Career strategy pertains to the individual's general approach to the realization of career goals and to the specificity of the goals themselves.
- Career tactics are actions to maintain oneself in a satisfactory employment situation.

The outcome of successful career management should include personal fulfillment, work-life balance, goal achievement, and financial security.

DEVELOPING GOALS

The career management process begins with setting goals. A relatively specific goal should first be formulated. This may be quite difficult when individuals lack knowledge of career opportunities and/or are not fully aware of their talents and abilities. Using career assessments may be a critical step in identifying opportunities and career paths that most resonate with the individual. Career assessments can range from quick and informal to more in-depth ones. Most assessments can be found on the Internet and are free, but they may not offer an in-depth evaluation.

Achievement of goals is based on time factors, and each type has a major influence on the formulation:

1. ***Short-term goals***, implemented over a 1- or 2-year period, are usually specific and limited in scope. Short-term goals are easier to formulate. Make sure they are achievable and relate to longer-term career goals.
2. ***Intermediate goals***, implemented over 3 to 5 years, tend to be less specific and more open ended than short-term goals. Both intermediate and long-term goals are more difficult to formulate than short-term goals because there are so many unknowns about the future.
3. ***Long-term goals***, developed and implemented more than 5 years in the future, are the most fluid of all. Lack of life experience and knowledge about potential opportunities and pitfalls make the formulation of long-term goals very difficult. These goals, however, may be easily modified as additional information is received without a great loss of career efforts because of experience/knowledge transfer from one career to another.

Because of the changing nature of the needs of organizations, individuals have to revisit the aforementioned process more frequently both now and in the future to maintain and enhance their employability. According to Schreuder and Coetzee (2006), an individual's decision to join an organization may depend on any of 3 factors: the objective factor, the subjective factor, and critical contact.

- **The objective factor model** assumes that the applicants are rational. The choice, then, is exercised after an objective assessment of the tangible benefits of the job. Factors evaluated include salary, other benefits, location, and opportunities for career advancement.
- **The subjective factor model** suggests that decision making is dominated by social and psychological factors. The status of the job, reputation of the organization, and other similar factors play an important role.

- **The critical contact model** advances the idea that a candidate's observations while interacting with the organization play a vital role in decision making. For example, how the recruiter keeps in touch with the candidate, the promptness of response, and similar factors are important. This model is more valid with experienced professionals.

These models assume that candidates have a free choice of employers and careers. In reality, the scarcity of jobs and the presence of strong competition for desirable jobs severely skew the decision-making process. In many instances, employees work particular careers simply because they were forced to accept whatever work was available to them. In addition, it has been found that culture can have a major influence on career choice (Ott-Holland, Huang, Ryan, Elizondo, & Wadlington, 2013).

When a person chooses a career that is best fit, there are multiple things to consider. According to an article in *U.S. World and News Report* by Tyrell-Smith (2010), these include natural talents, work style, social interaction, work-life balance, whether or not the person is looking to give back, whether the person is comfortable in the public eye, whether the person comfortably deals with stress or not, and, finally, how much money can be made. If choosing a career feels like too much pressure, another option is to pick a path that feels right today by making the best decision possible, knowing that a change could be made in the future. In today's workplace, choosing a career does not necessarily mean sticking with that line of work for a lifetime. After making a smart decision, plan to reevaluate down the line based on long-term objectives.

THE PROCESS OF CAREER PLANNING

The process of career planning is also known as career development. These steps are used to help plan a future career:

1. **Self-assessment**—is a process that helps assess the person's skills, potential, strengths, and ability to fulfill predetermined aims. As the name of the step suggests, the person assesses himself or herself and then, based on identified strengths and weaknesses, drafts a future plan. Executing this step helps to finalize the profession and career path the person wants to choose. It is probably best to choose and finalize more than one career, in case the first choice is not attainable.
2. **Self-development**—requires identifying what qualities and skills are necessary to help achieve the aims and goals previously established. For instance, the person might decide that he or she needs training or particular academic coursework in a field to be prepared for the chosen profession.

3. **Thorough job research**—requires the person to identify, through intensive researching, what career options and skills are necessary to succeed. The following questions should be answered:
   a. What is the scope of the chosen career?
   b. Will that career pay off in the future?
   c. Is there room for expansion in that career field?
4. **Create an action plan**—by translating the plans on a document. This step requires the person to identify how to achieve and fulfill the steps already decided. The best way to come up with an action plan is to come up with small goals that can be easily attained.
5. **Action**—to begin implementing the plan. The person should keep a very close eye on all activities to make sure that following this path will result in the achievement of the goal.

PLANNING BY HEALTH CARE ORGANIZATIONS

With more job vacancies expected and fewer workers available to fill them, health care organizations are pressured to discover new ways to fill critical jobs as well as find ways to retain productive workers. Internal development strategies for current employees provide one solution. However, some employers avoid investing adequate time and money for training and development fearing that employees, once trained, will leave their current employment with their new skills. When researching future careers, candidates should seek organizations that provide opportunities for career growth, learning, and development. Health care organizations should understand that these opportunities for career growth provide a very important recruiting and retention strategy (Wagner, 2000). In fact, a study by the Hay Group (2001) demonstrated that there is a correlation between job satisfaction, career development, and retention of employees. Thus, organizations should focus on the career development of existing employees to improve job satisfaction in this era of institutional change and growth. This strategy is an essential activity to remain competitive and survive in this dynamically changing industry.

Management development plays an important role in retaining staff through the process of leadership development, which provides growth opportunities for high-performing employees seeking management positions. Surveys have indicated that many employees harbor negative feelings toward their managers' abilities, underscoring the importance of management development to a retention strategy (Gering & Conner, 2002). Management positions in hospitals are usually filled within the current work group because a manager's technical qualifications generally need to mirror those in the department (McConnell, 2002). Unfortunately, what often occurs within the nursing field is that leaders are promoted into management roles out of need rather than because they have clearly demonstrated the skills and capacity necessary for managers. However, clinical work excellence is a poor predictor of management or leadership success. Therefore, retaining managers promoted in this fashion has been a chronic failure. Therefore, management development training should be included in a career ladder or path for select professionals within the department or discipline.

SUCCESSION PLANNING

With demand for health care services growing at such a rapid pace, health care organizations have to prepare for future workforce needs in many service areas. Traditional workforce and succession plans usually focus on job titles and duties already existing in the organization. The problem with this methodology is the focus on historical data rather than on future or strategic data. To achieve optimal results, workforce planning must be tied to the strategic plan of the organization (Guinn, 2000). As an example, a traditional unit in a hospital may be composed of a clinical director, unit coordinator, several charge nurses, and several dozen nursing employees. In the future, there may be a strategic initiative to grow the unit, adding clinical specialists, educators, physical therapists, caseworkers, and a larger staff of nursing personnel. Organizations focused on history as a planning guide will not have an accurate picture of competencies needed and are more likely to train or hire for positions no longer in existence. The forward-thinking organization will forecast the skills needed in the future, such as managers and staff better prepared for changes in technology or higher-level job functions.

Future leaders must have the ability to work with diverse groups of people, be able to adapt to change, and have strong critical thinking skills. For the person considering a career path in health care management, it would be necessary to ensure that these skills were learned before taking on these responsibilities. Another career path where the person is seeking career progression could be pursuing a position in a specialty area or higher-level skill set as opposed to a management position. One example is seeking experience, skill, and certification as a critical care nurse or an advanced practice nurse such as a nurse practitioner. And further progression for these employees would be considering a practice doctorate, such as the Doctor of Nursing Practice, or, if the employee wanted to move into a research-based position, a Doctor of Philosophy in nursing or another related field.

Today, nurses are being recruited for positions outside of traditional nursing and clinical areas. Nurses are filling positions in the pharmaceutical industry, insurance industry, case management firms, and legal firms, just to name a few. The nurse should do research into areas that seem attractive and compare and contrast his or her own knowledge and skill set with that of a career that might be of interest outside the walls of traditional nursing.

USING A CAREER COUNSELOR

The primary role of the career counselor is to meet with an individual to discuss current and projected needs in a field of interest to the individual. At this initial stage, an assessment of the existing need and the projected need would be done. If additional training is needed or required, then an assessment of local colleges and universities would be done to identify formal education. And in this day and age of technology, the career counselor can also evaluate programs anywhere in the United States or, for that matter, anywhere in the world. The career counselor would then identify the demand for an employee with the required new training. The career counselor would also assist in identifying tuition and scholarship programs to assist the individual in formulating a financial plan while obtaining the necessary credentials.

USING A MENTOR

Mentoring is defined as the process of experts facilitating learning through workplace interactions that allow the learner to construct his or her own knowledge and understanding with a goal of promoting the protégé's career development (Grindel, 2003). Even though the benefits of mentoring may be residual, when mentoring is done correctly, the result should match the main goals of the career development program. The mentor can be an executive, a manager, a coworker in the desired position or level, or a person outside of the area where the employee works. The mentor takes on the role of guide, advisor, coach, sponsor, motivator, and role model during these processes (Grindel, 2003). The relationship between the mentor and protégé during the learning process provides both instrumental and psychological components for success. The instrumental component supplies the necessary knowledge, and the psychological component provides feedback, which gives the protégé support in a nonthreatening manner. The key to a mentoring program is having mentors who are subject matter experts and who have additional training in the mentoring process. When choosing a mentor, careful consideration must be made to make sure that the mentor is appropriate and in the right position to be able to assist and has the resources—time and emotional and intellectual capabilities—to dedicate to the relationship (Doody, 2003).

CONCLUSION

Having the right career can be a source of great pride. It provides a positive self-image and sense of accomplishment. It determines where you live and who your friends are and largely determines your standard of living. When determining which career path to follow, things to consider are your personality, your interests, your skills, your life's goals, and, most importantly, current job trends.

As an alternative, it is important to also mention the phenomenon of serendipity—being in the right place at the right time. In a personal communication with Dr. Gloria Donnelly (2017), Dean Emerita of Drexel University College of Nursing and Health Professions in Philadelphia, Pennsylvania, this author discussed serendipity, which might very well occur more often than one thinks. In fact, both Dr. Donnelly and this author have relied completely on serendipity as the process of progressive career choices. The take-away here is, in addition to formal career development paths, be keenly aware of what is going on around you. You may "accidentally" walk easily into the very career you wanted.

QUESTIONS

1. The largest demographic group in the United States is the:
   a. Millennials
   b. Generation Xs
   c. Baby boomers
   d. Depression-era generation
2. The process of selecting career goals and the path to accomplish those goals is:
   a. Career planning
   b. Career orientation
   c. Career tactics
   d. Career strategy
3. Successful career management should include:
   a. Personal fulfillment
   b. Work-life balance
   c. Financial security
   d. All of the above
4. The goals that are usually specific and limited in scope are called:
   a. Short-term goals
   b. Intermediate goals
   c. Long-term goals
   d. Objective goals

5. If the individual's decision to join an organization relies on the status of the job and the reputation of the organization, the individual would be following:
   a. The objective factor model
   b. The subjective factor model
   c. The critical contact model
   d. None of the above
6. Workforce planning that is tied to the strategic plan of the organization is known as:
   a. Management development
   b. Recruitment strategies
   c. Succession planning
   d. Career planning

ANSWERS: 1-c, 2-a, 3-d, 4-a, 5-b, 6-c

References

Dictionary.reference.com. (Accessed 15 July 2017).

Donnelly, G. (2017). Personal communication.

Doody, M. F. (2003). A mentor is a key to career success. *Healthcare Financial Management, 57*(2), 92–93.

Gering, J., & Conner, J. (2002). A strategic approach to employee retention. *Healthcare Financial Management, 56*(11), 40–44.

Grindel, C. G. (2003). Mentoring managers. *Nephrology Nursing Journal, 30*(5), 517–522.

Guinn, S. L. (2000). Succession planning without job titles. *Career Development International, 5*(7), 390–394.

McConnell, C. R. (2002). The health care professional as a manager: Finding the critical balance in a dual role. *The Health Care Manager, 20*(3), 1–10.

Ott-Holland, C. J., Huang, J. L., Ryan, A. M., Elizondo, F., & Wadlington, P. L. (2013). Culture and vocational interests: The moderating role of collectivism and gender equalitarianism. *Journal of Counseling Psychology, 60*(4), 569–581. doi: 10.1037/a0033587.

Randstad North America, L. P. (2000). *Randstad North American employee review*. Atlanta: Brochure.

Schreuder, A. M. G., & Coetzee, M. (2006). *Careers: An organizational perspective*. Lansdowne Cape Town: Juta and Company Ltd.

The Hay Group. (2001). *Engage employees and boost performance*. Hay Group, Working Paper. Retrieved from www.haygroup.com.

Tyrell-Smith, T. (2010). *How to choose a career that's best for you. US News & World Report.*

Wagner, S. (2000). Retention: Finders, keepers. *Training and Development, 54*(8), 64.

Werther, W. B., & Davis, K. (1993). *Human resources and personnel management* (4th ed.). New York: McGraw-Hill Inc.

CHAPTER

12

Succession Planning

Virginia "Ginny" Wilson

This chapter will review:

LEADER COMPETENCIES IN SUCCESSION PLANNING

MENTORING IN SUCCESSION PLANNING

STRATEGIES FOR SUCCESSION PLANNING AND LEADERSHIP DEVELOPMENT

THE SUCCESSION PLAN

Nurse leaders play a key role in preparing an organization and the workforce for an inevitable transition of leadership. Their role responsibilities include identifying others with leadership potential, beginning with the recruitment and hiring stage, improving internal bench strength, increasing diversity of candidate pools, sharing talent internally more efficiently, and increasing organizational flexibility and employee job satisfaction (Bondas, 2006; Kim, 2012; Titzer, Phillips, Tooley, Hall, & Shirey, 2013; Titzer & Shirey, 2013). This leadership competency of succession planning is recognized by the American Association of Nurse Executives as an essential competency to prepare organizations for the undeniable fact of upcoming leadership transition (AONE, 2015):

- Develop a leadership succession plan.
- Promote nursing leadership as a desirable specialty.
- Mentor current and future nurse leaders.
- Establish mechanisms that provide for early identification and mentoring of staff with leadership potential.
- Develop a workforce analysis plan and implement strategies to ensure an adequate and qualified workforce.

Health care organizations face marketplace challenges such as restructuring, mergers, acquisitions, and/or bankruptcy that threaten operations in light of a looming leadership crisis (Griffith, 2012; Hader, Saver, & Steltzer, 2006).

Succession planning provides a safety margin for the organization through a process that includes electing, developing, and retaining the members of an organization who have the skills needed to sustain and move the practice or organization forward.

Turnover for nurse executives can be a result of many factors, not the least of which include general aging, catastrophic events, illness, job satisfaction issues, or simply retirement. Succession planning is more than a replacement strategy. Succession planning recognizes that turnover is inevitable and provides a planned strategic approach to attract, retain, and develop the leadership talent within the organization. Nurse leaders are as much at risk for a leadership crisis in the ranks as any other industry. Hader et al. (2006) and Johnson and D'Argenio (1991) argue that a plan for succession is essential and should consist of the elements of preparation, education, and development. Without a succession plan in place, few organizations are fully prepared to continue operations with as little disruption as possible when leadership needs occur (McCallin, Bamford-Wade, & Frankson, 2009; Sverdlik, 2012).

Organizations with formal succession plans are better positioned to avoid disruption of direction and workflow while facing the unknown reimbursement economy. In addition to the reimbursement/political environment challenges, the average age of a nurse in the United States is a major factor in the consideration. Who will be ready to replace current leaders when the time comes? The argument of concern and time for action is supported in the evidence from the Department of Labor Bureau of Labor Statistics (2010) that notes "… Additionally, hundreds of thousands of job openings will result from the need to replace experienced nurses who leave the occupation." Preparation begins now with development, coaching, and hiring.

Succession planning requires a strategic plan and a clear vision with buy-in from all levels of the organization. Leadership development needs to be targeted to address not only today's needs of the organization but also future needs because health care delivery in organizations will continue to evolve based on the marketplace. An important component of the strategic plan is to develop as many people as possible who are willing and able, especially because the current perception of a nurse leader's job is not as positively viewed as it could be (Huston, 2008; Wendler, Olson-Sitki, & Prater, 2009).

Succession planning as a strategic initiative has added benefits for the operations of the organization. The literature supports the fact that organizations with succession plans in place find increased employee job satisfaction, greater efficiency in talent sharing, and an overall increase organizational flexibility (Griffith, 2012).

Nurse leaders drive the succession planning process by being active in developing real-time experiences for learners that help build leadership competencies, devoting the time and attention needed to plan leadership development, and dedicating the time and attention to planned leadership training. Nurse leaders are key for health care delivery organizations to be able to maintain high levels of safe, efficient, and quality services that include a smooth transition of leadership through succession planning. As a key business strategy, succession planning supports the organization's missions to deliver quality health care services and serves to protect the organization by developing future leadership replacement needs (Collins, 2001; Drenkard, 2010; Redman, 2006).

The literature addressing management and leadership has supported the required need for succession planning to support the work of an organization. Beginning with Fayol in 1916, organizations needed to plan for succession and leadership turnover to provide for continuity. Rothwell et al. (2005) expanded on Fayol's work arguing that Fayol identified basic generic needs that are required by every organization to protect the organization's core and continuity. Those efforts to address core and continuity require the development of talent and maintenance of a "bench" of prepared talent who are ready and able to assume the mantle of leadership when the need arises.

In addition to general commentary, early research into continuity and succession planning uncovered 4 themes that are still valid today when considering leader succession and evaluating an organization's sustainability and profitability. They include successor origin, organizational size and rate of succession, succession and postsuccession performance, and succession precursors, such as leadership style and organizational characteristics (Boeker, 1997; Gamson & Scotch, 1964; McTeer, White, & Persad, 1995). These 4 themes contribute to the cycle of input, process, and outcome when developing and executing a succession plan.

Although there is no real evidence that one size succession plan fits all, the message is clear that in a changing health care delivery landscape, the future success of health care delivery models lies in the ability to be prepared for leadership transition in an as smooth as possible process. This smooth changeover of leadership will support continuity of the organizational goals and mission and promote profitability for survival.

Best practices in succession planning begin with the commitment of the organization's leadership to grow their bench strength through leadership development. As a strategic initiative, the plan for succession planning embraces specific elements that include leveraging human capital, creating a culture of talent sharing, creating opportunities for education, and application and measurement through established metrics.

Creating the environment for the succession plan and development process requires a change in the culture. This new culture is transparent, is proactive in problem solving, and takes a reflective view of what is needed to support leadership development for the future.

Transparency supports the organization's ability to keep individuals with talent and reduce or eliminate replacement hiring. Transparency in this culture is practiced, not just talked about, by keeping things visible and open to all, and contributes to building trust. Trust requires that individuals have access to information, that there is consistency in what will constitute success in training and development, and, when there is opportunity for advancement, that there is honesty in the promotion/upward mobility processes.

Organizations practicing succession planning and leadership development keep the process and opportunities for leadership development transparent. This in turn leads to opportunities for additional mentorships and provides more transitional support into a leadership role (Groves, 2007; Rothwell, 2002, 2010).

In this culture of preparing for the future and succession planning, employees feel valued. As such, employees become valued stakeholders in the organization's achievement of its end goals and objectives. They become more engaged, participate actively, recognize a larger work group than just a nuclear one, and see the organization as a whole, leading to wider interaction among work groups.

Collins (2001) argues that linking training and development to action-oriented meaningful projects and initiatives leads to clockwork organizations, time ticking by but each minute maximized. Such clockwork organizations in industry are General Electric, Exxon-Mobil, Home Depot, and IBM, to name a few. The succession plan takes hold at the point of hire, and employees are groomed over a series of years to be ready to fulfill leadership roles when vacancies occur. Leadership transition, thanks to succession planning and leadership development, is a smooth transition and avoids disruption.

MENTORING AS A PART OF LEADERSHIP DEVELOPMENT IN SUCCESSION PLANNING

Mentoring is viewed as a mechanism to support leadership development, even given the title of an esteemed connection (McCloughen, O'Brien, & Jackson, 2009). The title of esteemed connection implies a special bond between 2 individuals, and indeed a mentor-mentee relationship is just that. In the formal sense, mentors not only work to transfer knowledge but also support and champion a mentee's development. Mentors are self-confident, competent, and committed to the development of others (McCloughen et al., 2009). Mentees have the advantage of observation and an interpersonal relationship with an experienced and established role model and as such will need to be self-directed, competent, and willing to learn.

Being a transformational leader contributes to the effectiveness of the mentoring process. Transformational leaders support a mentoring culture in which inspirational motivation, individualized consideration, idealized influence, and intellectual stimulations form the foundations for the interpersonal interactions (Bass, 1994). Just as with the concept of succession planning and leadership development, a mentoring culture requires executive support, flexibility, incentives, and recognition to be successful (Posey-Goodwin, 2013; Yamamura & Stedham, 2007).

Formal mentor programs may vary in structure and matching mentors with mentees. In developing the match, it is essential to have guidelines and parameters to avoid a mismatch for professional or interpersonal reasons (Simon & Eby, 2003). Mentoring will serve 2 functions: meeting career development needs and enhancing the mentee to learn what is needed for advancement as well as psychosocial function in providing acceptance, support, and encouragement (McCloughen et al., 2009; Tourigny & Pulich, 2005).

Informal mentoring as a part of leadership development is also evident and may have as important a role as formal mentoring programs (Downey, Parslow, & Smart, 2011; McCloughen et al., 2009). This unstructured relationship is built on the needs of the mentee and mentor and is not defined by purpose or by longevity. Informal leaders serve as mentors as they influence the culture by sharing their knowledge and expertise, exhibiting team behaviors, and genuinely caring for others.

Formal and informal mentoring are often considered face to face, but as the world grows smaller and technology supports learning and experiences there is room to consider e-mentoring (de Janasz, Ensher, & Heun, 2008; Pietsch & Williamson, 2010). Industries already use e-mentoring for real-time interaction when a live mentor is not available, enhancing communication and learning. Although there is no literature available to evaluate the effectiveness of e-mentoring for nurse leadership development, the concept is as enticing as the use of technology in all others facets of life, providing the right information at the right time. Mentoring in all iterations requires resources and time that organizations must support to be a successful component of succession planning and leadership development (Posey-Goodwin, 2013; Yamamura & Stedham, 2007).

BASIC STRATEGIES FOR SUCCESSION PLANNING AND LEADERSHIP DEVELOPMENT

Best practice organizations already provide a template that can be customized for each individual organization. Any succession plan must be flexible to accommodate the changing needs of the health care organization and industry. Anticipating the planned and natural turnover of leadership positions will direct the focus on the plan for leadership development programs. This will be a process for the whole organization, so the roles and responsibilities of everyone involved in the process must be spelled out.

Beginning with an assessment step, determine high performers, high potential, and current leader positions. Competencies flow from position descriptions and define work and job responsibilities. Nurse executive competencies can be found in the AONE (2005) and ANA (2016) literature, basically including the expectation that the leader is a skilled communicator and a change agent in a transformational leadership style.

In the early stages of succession and leadership development planning, there is an opportunity to consider adding leadership training that is geared to the interests of potential leaders in the form of classes, coaches, mentors, or new work assignments. Real-world learning and contemporary challenges make the learning more effective in translating classroom to the practice environment. Project-driven work creates an opportunity for learners and leaders to work together in the planning, development, execution, and evaluation of ventures that have a real-time impact on the organization and the learner.

A DEVELOPMENT PLAN FOR SUCCESSION

Creating a development plan that contains realistic goals, a description of the learning process and available support mechanisms, and how the learning can be used in the current work environment contributes to success. Within the organization there will need to be a plan for the process when leadership vacancies occur and how candidates will be selected from the new pool. Transparency is crucial when vacancies occur so that applicants know the process for advertising the vacancy and any limitations that may be a part of the vacancy opportunities. Communication is essential to be able to openly discuss with the candidate in private his or her readiness for the position or the need to continue in targeted areas of development.

Executing the plan for the first time will present challenges at the start, but as in all change, this effort will position a health care organization in a stronger survival position. Industry and business provide many examples of organizations that have thrived in challenging economic conditions. Part of that success can be seen rooted in their commitment to leadership development programs and building their bench strength with potential leadership candidates. Other organizations have set the standard for succession planning and leadership development and have proved that successful, sustainable, and profitable organizations support a culture that grows internal talent, and health care organizations are capable of repeating this success.

Lastly, everything ends with an evaluation loop, and it is essential to know how effective the plan and process have been. Because there is no one size fits all, each organization will need to determine what works and what does not to adjust and change the plan and programs. Just like plan-do-check-act, the A is ready and able to be adjusted. As with all performance improvement initiatives, the questions asked will provide the data necessary to make revisions that are unique to the individual organization. General evaluation questions may include how have the internal candidates, promoted, fit into their new roles, what is their success rate, and have the expectations met the realities of the need?

The overall impact on an organization once a succession plan is in place and leadership development is part of the culture includes knowledge acquisition, appreciation of knowledge, learning appraisals, application possibilities (current and future), process evaluation for effectiveness and efficiency, and a reward process for achievements. The evaluation loop keeps the process in alignment with the outcomes requirements and provides an opportunity to measure the success from building internal bench strength to prepare for the future leadership needs.

CONCLUSION

Succession planning and leadership development as a strategic initiative is the practice or an organization's process to see an end return on its investment, or sustainability and profitability. Succession planning and development is a sound approach to strategic management of an organization and reflects leaders who are competent in managing the climate, culture, and outcomes. Preparing nurses to transition from the clinical environment to being an effective leader with new and specialized knowledge requires training and development to promote with preparation and support leadership transition without disruption for the organization. Succession planning and talent development is an extension of who nurse leaders are. Using a known process of planning, developing, delivering, and evaluating, preparing for inevitable leadership turnover is a competency that nurse leaders embrace.

References

American Nurses Association. (2016). *Nursing administration: Scope and standards of nursing practice* (2nd ed.). Silver Spring, MD: American Nurses Publishing.

American Organization of Nurse Executives. (2015). *AONE nurse executive competencies.* Retrieved from http://www.aone.org/resources/nec.pdf.

Bass, B. M. (1994). *Improving organizational effectiveness through transformational leadership.* Thousand Oaks, CA: Sage Publications.

Boeker, W. (1997). Strategic change: The influence of managerial characteristics and organizational growth. *Academy of Management Journal, 40*(1), 152–170.

Bondas, T. (2006). Paths to nursing leadership. *Journal of Nursing Management, 14*(5), 332–339. Retrieved from CINAHL with Full Text database.

Collins, J. (2001). *Good to great.* New York, NY: Harper Business.

de Janasz, S. C., Ensher, E. A., & Heun, C. (2008). Virtual relationships and real benefits: Using e-mentoring to connect business students with practicing managers. *Mentoring & Tutoring: Partnership in Learning, 16*(4), 394–411.

Downey, M., Parslow, S., & Smart, M. (2011). The hidden gem in nursing leadership: Informal leaders. *Journal of Nursing Management, 19*, 517–521.

Drenkard, K. (2010). The business case for magnet. *JONA, 40*(6), 263–271.

Gamson, W., & Scotch, N. (1964). Scapegoating in baseball. *American Journal of Sociology, 70*, 69–72. Retrieved from JSTOR database.

Griffith, M. (2012). Effective succession planning in nursing: A review of the literature. *Journal of Nursing Management, 20*(14).

Groves, K. S. (2007). Integrating leadership development and succession planning best practices. *Journal of Management Development, 26*(3), 239–260.

Hader, R., Saver, C., & Steltzer, T. (2006). No time to lose. *Nursing Management, 37*(7), 23–48. Retrieved from Academic Search Premier database. Hall.

Huston, C. (2008). Preparing nurse leaders for 2020. *Journal of Nursing Management, 16*, 905–911.

Johnson, K. R., & D'Argenio, C. (1991). Management training effects on nurse manager leadership behavior. *Nursing Economics, 9*(4), 249–254. Retrieved from CINAHL with Full Text database.

Kim, T. H. (2012). Succession planning in hospitals and the association with organizational performance. *Nursing Economics, 30*, 14–20.

McCallin, A., Bamford-Wade, A., & Frankson, C. (2009). Leadership succession planning: A key issue for the nursing profession. *Nurse Leader, 7*(6), 40–44.

McCloughen, A., O'Brien, L., & Jackson, D. (2009). Esteemed connection: Creating a mentoring relationship for nurse leadership. *Nursing Inquiry, 16*(4), 326–336.

McTeer, W., White, P. G., & Persad, S. (1995). Manager/coach mid-season replacement and team performance in professional team sport. *Journal of Sport Behavior, 18*(1), 58–68.

Pietsch, M., & Williamson, J. (2010). "Getting the pieces together": Negotiating the transition from pre-service to in-service teacher. *Asia-Pacific Journal of Teacher Education, 38*(4), 331–344.

Posey-Goodwin. (2013). Exploring preferences of mentoring activities among Generational Groups of Registered Nurses in Florida. (Doctoral dissertation). Retrieved from ProQuest, LLC. (Accession No. ED553007).

Redman, R. (2006). Leadership succession planning: an evidence-based approach for managing the future. *JONA*, *36*(6), 292–297.

Rothwell, W. J. (2002). Putting success into your succession planning. *Journal of Business Strategy*, *23*(3), 32–37.

Rothwell, W. J. (2010). *Effective succession planning: Ensuring leadership continuity and building talent from within.* New York: American Management Association.

Rothwell, W. J., Wang, W. A., Jackson, R. D., Payne, T. D., Knight, S., & Lindholm, J. E. (2005). *Career planning and succession management: Developing your organizations talent - for today and tomorrow*. Westport, CT: Praegar.

Simon, S. A., & Eby, L. T. (2003). A typology of negative mentoring experience: A multidimensional scaling study. *Human Relations*, *56*(9), 1083–1106.

Sverdlik, B. (2012). Who will be our nursing leaders in the future? The role of succession planning. *Journal of Nursing Administration*, *42*(7/8), 383–385.

Titzer J., Phillips, T., Tooley, S., Hall, N., & Shirey, M. (2013). Nurse manager succession planning: Synthesis of the evidence. *Journal of Nursing Management*, *21*(7), 971–979.

Titzer, J. L. & Shirey, M. R. (2013). Nurse manager succession planning: A concept analysis. *Nursing Forum*, *48*, 155–164.

Tourigny, L., & Pulich, M. (2005). A critical examination of formal and informal mentoring among nurses. *The HealthCare Manager*, *24*(1), 68–76.

United States Department of Labor, Bureau of Labor Statistics (2010). Retrieved from http://www.bls.gov/oco/ocos083.htm.

Wendler, M. C., Olson-Sitki, K., & Prater, M. (2009). Succession planning for RNs: Implementing a nurse management internship. *Journal of Nursing Administration*, *39*(7/8), 326–333.

Yamamura, J., & Stedham, Y. (2007). Gender differences in business ethics: justice and relativist perspectives. *Business Ethics: A European Review*, *16*(2), 163–164.

CHAPTER 13

Technology Tips for the Nurse Executive

Mary Gallagher Gordon

This chapter will review:

ELECTRONIC MEDICAL RECORDS—TECHNOLOGY USE, SECURITY, AND CONTINGENCY PLANS

MEANINGFUL USE

SYSTEMS AND THE END USER

HIPAA AND SOCIAL MEDIA PRINCIPLES

In today's health care, technology is incorporated into many aspects of the day-to-day workflow. It has replaced the paper, pens, and filing cabinets of the 1990s. Yet there is still much to be done with technology integration in health care, and it is essential for the nurse executive to understand, embrace, and champion for continual technology improvements in all aspects of the health care area. For example, did you know that the typical online banking system times out when your computer is idle for 7 minutes? What is the timeout for the computers at the current facility? Longer? Why? Why are we protecting our money and not our patient's health care information? As a nursing executive, the ability to have knowledge at one's fingertips, to find information to make informed decisions, and to surround oneself with those who have the expertise in health care informatics will be an asset. The American Organization of Nurse Executives (AONE) has 7 competencies related to health care informatics, whereas the American Nurses Credentialing Center (ANCC) has 4 sections with technology content threaded throughout. These competencies have been assimilated in this chapter to better prepare the nurse executive for the changes that are constantly affecting health care technology.

Historically, technology changes took off in 2004, with the then President, George Bush, urging the U.S. health care facilities to move from paper to electronic charting within 10 years. In 2009 the American Reinvestment and Recovery Act was passed, which included technology measures such as the Health Information Technology for Economic and Clinical Health (HITECH) Act. The HITECH Act supports electronic patient information and a national health care technology network, a national goal. Meaningful use is defined as the use of the electronic health record (EHR) in a manner that assures the technology is connected and safely affords the ability to access information. Meaningful use comprises 5 pillars of health outcome priorities, including improvement of quality, safety, efficiency, and reducing health disparities; engaging patients in their care while having access to their health information; improving care coordination; improving population and public health; and ensuring adequate privacy and security of the patient's health information (CDC, 2017). For example, if the client who is seeing a primary care provider within your health care system became ill and was seen at a different facility within the same system, the EHR would pull out the client's most recent health information. Divided into 3 stages for facilities to meet in order to qualify for incentives, meaningful use commenced with data capturing and sharing during 2011 to 2012. During stage 1, there were 3 areas to be measured. The first area included 15 core set measures established to ensure standardized data entry within the areas of patient demographics, computerized physician order entry allergies, active medication list, problem lists, and recording of vital signs and documenting smoking status for those older than 15 years. The second area was 24 measures, of which 19 had to be met, including patient education and medication reconciliation. The third area was the integration of clinical quality measures, including hypertension, preventative care, and childhood immunization (AHRQ, 2013). Stage 2 was implemented in 2014 with a goal to advance clinical processes such as online access for patients to view their health information. The foundation of clinical decision support was started with stage 1, and stage 2 builds upon this with computerized physician order entry for all care, tracking medications via an electronic medication record, and recording smoking for those older than 13 years. Both stages 1 and 2 require that the health facility attest that they are meeting the mandatory measures of meaningful use (ONC, 2015). Stage 3 was optional in 2017 but is mandatory for 2018, with striving for better-quality outcomes to show improvements in the clients who are served. Specific measures are mandatory, and others are optional to qualify for federal funding. The Center for Medicare and Medicaid Services EHR incentive plan was put in place with the intent that hospitals would use the EHR in meaningful ways to receive federal funding (ONC, 2015). Meaningful use threads with the clinical quality measures used to ensure that the facility is providing safe, quality care to qualify for the EHR incentives (AHRQ, 2013). These measures are based on the 6 domains of health care quality, safe, effective, efficient, patient-centered, equitable, and timely care, as described in the 2001 Institute of Medicine report *Crossing the Quality Chasm: A New Health System for the 21st Century*:

- **Safe**: Avoiding harm to patients from the care that is intended to help them.
- **Effective**: Providing services based on scientific knowledge to all who could benefit and refraining from providing services to those not likely to benefit (avoiding underuse and misuse, respectively).
- **Patient centered**: Providing care that is respectful of and responsive to individual patient preferences, needs, and values and ensuring that patient values guide all clinical decisions.
- **Timely**: Reducing waits and sometimes harmful delays for both those who receive and those who give care.
- **Efficient**: Avoiding waste, including waste of equipment, supplies, ideas, and energy.
- **Equitable**: Providing care that does not vary in quality because of personal characteristics, such as gender, ethnicity, geographic location, and socioeconomic status (IOM, 2001).

Critical to the success of health care technology, as a leader, the nurse executive will need to critically evaluate the technology landscape to see where the facility is and where it should go related to these 6 domains. While establishing new technology, a comprehensive vision for a robust EMR should include the identified key stakeholders, end users, impact on workaround, redesign, integration into legacy systems, financial constraints, ethical considerations, and the impact on patients and families. Technology integration requires buy-in from the top-down with champions from all aspects of the facility. Workflow changes and the redesigns that will occur from the new technology need to be evaluated to allow safe and quality care to be delivered. Commitment to superusers and information technology (IT) support during the transition are critical to the success of the integration of the technology. If the decision is made to use one of the current large EMR vendors, it would be ideal to request to speak to a facility currently using the product and see what works and what does not work. What were the lessons learned during the transition from the old system to the new system, and could the identified challenges be avoided with the next EMR integration? Does the system allow for changes, integration of new care process models, and additional notifications? Will the current infrastructure work with the new EMR, or will a new infrastructure be integrated? In many health care facilities, there are different platforms where key technologies reside and there needs to be an ability to integrate the main components in the new EMR system. Follow-up on any issues, improvements, and updates must continue after implementation (Crosson et al., 2011). Human factors research is also critical to the implementation of new technology. As new systems are introduced, the potential for a near miss, actual errors that may be a system or human error, should be anticipated and discussed with the staff who will be affected by the changes with new technology. The culture of the health care facility should be one of a just culture, holding all accountable but responding in a fair and just way with each critical incident and error prevention.

Review of compliance criteria to understand if the EHR meets the Health Insurance Portability and Accountability Act (HIPAA) requirements is critical. The standards are by either an expert determination method or by safe harbor. The expert determination method is the use of acceptable statistical and scientific principles to deidentify the health information. Safe harbor is the deidentification of 18 protected health information (PHI) identifiers so that they cannot be traced back to protect patient identity. These 18 identifiers include the following:

1. Names
2. All geographic subdivisions smaller than a state, including street address, city, county, precinct, ZIP code, and their equivalent geocodes, except for the initial 3 digits of the ZIP code if, according to the current publicly available data from the Bureau of the Census:
   a. The geographic unit formed by combining all ZIP codes with the same 3 initial digits contains more than 20,000 people and
   b. The initial 3 digits of a ZIP code for all such geographic units containing 20,000 or fewer people is changed to 000
3. All elements of dates (except year) for dates that are directly related to an individual, including birth date, admission date, discharge date, death date, and all ages over 89 years and all elements of dates (including year) indicative of such age, except that such ages and elements may be aggregated into a single category of age 90 years or older
4. Telephone numbers
5. Vehicle identifiers and serial numbers, including license plate numbers
6. Fax numbers
7. Device identifiers and serial numbers
8. Email addresses
9. Web universal resource locators
10. Social Security numbers
11. Internet Protocol addresses

12. Medical record numbers
13. Biometric identifiers, including finger and voice prints
14. Health plan beneficiary numbers
15. Full-face photographs and any comparable images
16. Account numbers
17. Any other unique identifying number, characteristic, or code, except that the covered entity may assign a code or other means of record identification to allow information de-identified under this section to be re-identified by the covered entity, provided that: (a) *Derivation*. The code or other means of record identification is not derived from or related to information about the individual and is not otherwise capable of being translated so as to identify the individual; and (b) *Security*. The covered entity does not use or disclose the code or other means of record identification for any other purpose, and does not disclose the mechanism for re-identification.
18. Certificate/license numbers (HHS, 2015)

Does the EHR system's log-on require 2-factor authentication (2FA)? Although the HIPAA regulations do not explicitly spell out the requirements for 2FAs, the law does require an EHR system that protects patient data. Having the end user log on via a multiple authentication process may help meet the goal to keep the data secure. 2FA requires both a password and secondary credential, such as a biometric or personal identification number. Having an authentication system that does not require multiple passwords would be ideal. In addition, one must evaluate if the authentication system is efficient and effective to use.

Education on acceptable use is critical to the success of protection of the system. How are the end users educated about avoidance of phishing and the use of social media? Phishing is the act of getting an end user to disclose and share personal information typically after clicking on a link that will allow for the capturing of the data in a fraudulent manner (Christensson, 2006). Education about when to click and when not to click on links within emails is critical. According to Hay Newman (2017) there are 3 steps one should use to avoid a phishing attack. First, think twice before clicking on a link; consider the source of the email and then what is the plan if you do get phished. Second, review the email, whom it is from, and what the email address is; hover over the link, does it show where it is going? When working with the IT team within the facility, verify what tools are in place for email filters, scanning for spam, and plan what action should be taken if an employee is caught in a phishing incident. Third, staff need to understand who the IT staff are and how the IT staff would reach out to them if remote access to their computer is needed. More and more people are connected by multiple devices, and as a result the ability to connect with their social networks is typically close at hand. Social media include but are not limited to Twitter, Facebook, a blog, and any Internet platform that allows someone to post information. Therefore, a policy should be in place to address social media and the health care employee. An excellent resource is the American Nurses Association (ANA, 2011) fact sheet on navigating the world of social media. The 6 principles are as follows:

1. Nurses must not transmit or place online individually identifiable patient information.
2. Nurses must observe ethically prescribed professional patient-nurse boundaries.
3. Nurses should understand that patients, colleagues, institutions, and employers may view postings.
4. Nurses should take advantage of privacy settings and seek to separate personal and professional information online.
5. Nurses should bring content that could harm a patient's privacy, rights, or welfare to the attention of appropriate authorities.
6. Nurses should participate in developing institutional policies governing online conduct (ANA, 2011).

In addition to these 6 social media principles is the development of penalties if the policy was violated. Some facilities have established a no tolerance policy of use of social media while at work, whereas others may have a social media policy that the employee must sign. Using these 6 criteria in the development of a policy alongside of legal counsel input may be helpful. The nurse executive needs to remember that, in addition to the facility penalties, there may be federal regulators that would need to be notified if there was a social media incident with PHI. As a result, the nurse leader needs to be knowledgeable about ethics as related to technology. As McGonigle and Garver Mastrian (2018) stated, the goal of any system is that ethical decisions are reached, which are justified, rational, and follow standards of practice. The ANA Code of Ethics (2015) Provision 3 states that "the nurse promotes, advocates for, and strives to protect the health, safety, and rights of the patient." Knowledge of the compliance and education surrounding Internet use on hospital technology, use of social media, and phishing can help meet this ANA provision.

Does the system have encryption at rest as well as in transit? Encryption is the process of converting text into a coded text. Encryption tools allow the data to be put into an encoded text that requires a key to unlock and allow the receiver to read it. This process occurs both when the data are in transit and when the data are at rest. Data at rest are the data that are housed on the individual computer, flash drive, or system. Data in transit are the data that are in motion, moving from one location to another, either within the system or outside the system. For example, data in transit would be the sharing of the patient file between the hospital and the satellite office where the patient visits the primary doctor. Encryption of the technology systems is important for both data at rest and data in transit. For example, mobile devices, such as intravenous pumps, wearable technology, handheld computer tablets, or wireless printers, are at risk of getting hacked, as each mobile device that connects to the wireless system has the capability to expose the wireless facility system to vulnerabilities. How often are these systems getting updated? Working with vendors, the Chief Nursing Informatics Officer (CNIO), and the IT team to eradicate any potential vulnerabilities in the overall system is critical to the success of encryption.

What about backup for the EHR system? How often is a backup performed, and where are the backups stored? Is there redundancy? Is the backup cloud based or server based? What is the backup plan if the system shuts down? How often is the backup recovery system tested to be sure it is functional? The HIPAA Security Rule has been set up to ensure the confidentiality, integrity, and availability of EHR. The rule contains guidelines that both the covered entity and the business associate must follow for the protection of the PHI that may be received, maintained, or transmitted to avoid any cyberattacks (ONC, 2015). These safeguards requirements for an EHR contingency plan include a data backup plan, a disaster recovery plan, an emergency mode operations plan, and testing and revision of the procedures related to these plans. The data backup plan requires a plan for redundancy and storing of EHR copies. The disaster recovery plan is a plan to recover the lost data. Emergency mode operations plan allows for health care to continue during the emergency. Testing of these plans is critical to success in an emergency situation (OIG, 2016). In 2016 the Office of the Inspector General found that 95% of the hospitals had a contingency plan in place (Durben Hirsch, 2016). The need for a disaster recovery process is critical for the patients and the facility. This should include asset management of the technology within the facility, identification of potential vulnerable areas of the facility, and the impact on the facility if the recovery process could not be successfully implemented.

Is there the ability to perform audit logs, to ensure that only the providers that are delivering care are the only ones accessing the EHR for the client? This is a measurable component of stage 2 meaningful use under the HITECH Act (Pema, 2014). A plan should be in place for scheduled audits to assess that only people who need to access patient files are actually the only people who are accessing the files. In addition, random audits may be necessary if the facility had a client who was well known, such as a star sports player or actor, admitted. Ensuring that the system meets all compliance criteria is critical to patient's hospital security. How does one gather and retain all of this information? Research, read, and surround oneself with experts in key areas to support and assist with oversight of the technology within the health care facility.

While looking at this snapshot of IT requirements, the nurse executive should be a leader who embraces collaboration. Collaboration and the need to be inclusive are critical to the success of technology integration. Because nurses are one of the most frequent users of the EHR systems as well as mobile technology, looking for a CNIO within the leadership team would be ideal. Nursing informatics is the combination of the science of nursing with the integration of technology to take data and construct them into knowledge with the focus to advance patient care and quality within the health care environment (McGonigle, Hunter, Spies, & Hebda, 2014). The CNIO can engage with the nursing staff, collaborate with the chief medical informatics officer, and build an interprofessional team to align the mission and goals of the health care facility with technology integration (Kirby, 2015). These teams will need to be divided up depending on the amount of work that must be completed to meet all of the EHR requirements and security of the systems. Because staff nurses tend to be one of the heaviest users of the EHR, they must be included in the sustainability of systems, the process, and workflow changes with any implementation of new technology. Educating nurses within the clinical area on how technology can assist with the heavy lifting both with the delivery of quality patient care as well as workflow process. Educating nurses on how to take the data generated and process into information is a key skill set (McGonigle et al., 2014). Having a CNIO or a nurse leader who is well versed in informatics will help facilitate this process and allow the voice of the patient to be heard (Simpson, 2013).

For the nurse executive, the ability to understand statistical analysis to measure performance and change is ideal as is the ability to monitor quality improvement projects and the data generated to deliver quality care (Spath, 2009). Translating all of the health care data that are generated to meaningful information is a skill that the nurse executive should acquire. This leads to evidence-based practice to enhance overall processes within the facility. One will be required to write reports and describe the information in a meaningful way to the end users, and not causing information overload is critical. If one does a web search, the peer reviewed research on big data, data analytics as well as the ability to utilize de-identified health information can assist the nurse executive in learning how to write reports that show the impact of healthcare indicators identified.

Technology has come to the forefront of health care, and the nurse executive needs to know critical elements of the technology as well as surround oneself with those who are experts in the field. This must be done to continue to meet the needs of the clients served as well as the regulations and needs of the facility.

QUESTIONS

1. In 2009 the American Reinvestment and Recovery Act was passed, which included many technology measures such as:
   a. Affordable Care Act
   b. National Health Care Act
   c. Health Information Technology for Economic and Clinical Health Act
   d. Healthy Americans Act
2. Meaningful use utilizes quality indicators based on which 6 domains of health care?
   a. Efficient, family centered, effective, timely, equitable, and safe
   b. Family centered, costly, efficient, timely, safe, and equitable
   c. Effective, efficient, patient centered, equitable, safe, and timely care
   d. Equitable, costly, population centered, efficient, safe, and timely
3. With the integration of new technology, the nurse executive must be sure to include which of the following (select all that apply)?
   a. Workflow changes
   b. Self-paced usage
   c. Champions from only end users
   d. Commitment of IT and superusers on site
   e. Follow-up and updates after implementation
4. The nurse executive decides to use the expert determination method to maintain the EHR to meet HIPAA. Expert determination method is defined as:
   a. Geometry and math principles
   b. Statistical and scientific principles
   c. Deidentification of the 18 PHI criteria
   d. Device identifiers and serial numbers
5. When logging on to the hospital system, the nurse executive must use a 2FA and log in using:
   a. Biometric, user name, and/or password
   b. Office key and password
   c. Personal identification number and office key
   d. Credit card number and biometric
6. When reviewing social media, the nurse executive developed a social media policy that all staff members would sign. Included in this policy would be (select all that apply):
   a. Staff can transmit PHI to a social media online Web site
   b. Staff should separate work from social online information
   c. Staff should realize that other staff may see social postings
   d. Staff should not bring posts that may have patient information to administration
7. Encryption of PHI is important. This includes (select all that apply):
   a. Data at rest
   b. Data in transit
   c. Data on desktops
   d. Data moving from the hospital to the office

8. The HIPAA Security Rule has been set up to ensure the confidentiality, integrity, and availability of EHR. The safeguard requirements for this rule include:
   a. An EHR contingency plan
   b. Onboarding plan
   c. General mode operation plan
   d. Data plan
9. Collaboration is critical to the success of technology integration. Key to this is a CNIO, as this person (select all that apply):
   a. Brings the science of nursing and technology to take data and construct to knowledge
   b. Can be the voice of nursing and the clients served
   c. Will monopolize the technical team
   d. Build interprofessional teams
10. The nurse executive knows that knowledge comes from analyzing data and translating it to meaningful information. One of the goals of this knowledge is:
    a. Generating more reports
    b. Increasing workload for staff
    c. Development of evidence-based practice
    d. Changing the mission statement

ANSWERS: 1-c, 2-c, 3-a, d, e, 4-b, 5-a, 6-b, c, 7-a, b, c, d, 8-a, 9-a, b, d, 10-c

References

AHRQ. (2013). *Practice facilitation handbook. Module 17. Electronic health records and meaningful use.* https://www.ahrq.gov/professionals/prevention-chronic-care/improve/system/pfhandbook/mod17.html.

American Nurses Association (ANA). (2011). *Fact sheet-navigating the world of social media.* www.nursingworld.org/FunctionalMenuCategories/AboutANA/Social-Media/Social-Networking-Principles-Toolkit/Fact-Sheet-Navigating-the-World-of-Social-Media.pdf+&cd=1&hl=en&ct=clnk&gl=us.

American Nurses Association (ANA). (2015). *Code of ethics for nurses with interpretive statements.* Silver Spring, MD: American Nurses Association.

American Nurses Credentialing Center (ANCC). http://nursecredentialing.org/NurseExecutive.

American Organization of Nurse Executives (AONE). http://www.aone.org/initiatives/cenp-prepare.shtml.

Center for Disease Control and Prevention. (2017). *Meaningful use.* https://www.cdc.gov/ehrmeaningfuluse/introduction.html.

Christensson, P. (2006). *Phishing definition.* Retrieved from https://techterms.com.

Crosson, J., Etz, R., Wu S., Strauss, S., Eisenman, D., & Bell, D. (2011). Meaningful use of electronic prescribing in 5 exemplar primary care practices. *Annuals of Family Medicine, 9*(5), 392–397.

Department of Health and Human Services Office of the Inspector General (OIG). (2016). *Hospitals largely reported addressing requirements for EHR contingency plans.* https://oig.hhs.gov/oei/reports/oei-01-14-00570.asp.

Durben Hirsch, M. (2016). *Hospitals 'largely' addressing HIPAA requirements for EHR contingency plans. FierceHealthcare.* http://www.fiercehealthcare.com/it/oig-hospitals-largely-addressing-hipaa-requirements-for-ehr-contingency-plans.

Hay Newman, L. (2017). *Phishing scams even fool tech nerds-here's how to avoid them. Wired.* https://www.wired.com/2017/03/phishing-scams-fool-even-tech-nerds-heres-avoid/.

Health and Human Services.gov (HHS). (2015). *Guidance regarding methods for de-identification of protected health information in accordance with the health insurance portability and accountability act (HIPAA) privacy rule.* https://www.hhs.gov/hipaa/for-professionals/privacy/special-topics/de-identification/index.html.

Institute of Medicine. (2001). *Crossing the quality chasm: A new health system for the 21st century.* Washington, DC: National Academy Press.

Kirby, S. (2015). Informatics leadership: The role of the CNIO. *Nursing.* doi:10.1097/01.NURSE.0000462394.23939.8e.

McGonigle, D., & Garver Mastrian, K. (2018). *Nursing informatics and the foundation of knowledge* (4th ed.). Burlington, MA: Jones and Bartlett Learning.

McGonigle, D., Hunter, K., Spies, C., & Hebda, T. (2014). Why nurses need to understand nursing informatics. *Association of Perioperative Registered Nurses (AORN) Journal, 100*(3), 324–327.

Pena, G. (2014). *Using big data to audit access to patient data and beyond. Healthcare Informatics.* https://www.healthcare-informatics.com/article/using-big-data-audit-access-patient-data-and-beyond.

Simpson, R. (2013). Chief nurse executives need contemporary informatics competencies. *Nursing Economic$, 31*(6), 277–287.

Spath, P. (2009). Role of HIM professionals in quality management. *Perspectives in Health Information Management*, 6(1). https://www.ncbi.nlm.nih.gov/pmc/articles/PMC2781733/.

The Office of the National Coordinator for Health Information Technology (ONC). (2015). *Guide to privacy and security of electronic health information.* HealthIT.gov.

APPENDIX

A

Nursing Executive: Certification Prep Questions

1. Responsibilities of the governing board of the hospital include all of the following **except**:
   a. Selecting a chief executive officer and delegating to him or her the authority to manage the hospital
   b. Assuring the hospital's short- and long-range financial stability
   c. Appointing the chief nurse executive as a voting member of the hospital board
   d. Communicating the goals and performance of the hospital to the community

2. Which of the following items do not pertain to ADA requirements for the work environment?
   a. Position descriptions
   b. Physical facilities
   c. Hiring practices
   d. Workmen's compensation policies

3. On your medical unit you are monitoring the following quality indicators:
   A. The registered nurse (RN) administers flu vaccines to patients who sign consent.
   B. At the time of discharge, the patient is provided with information on how to prevent infection in his or her surgical wound.

   Which of the following is the correct classification of these indicators (structure, process, outcome)?
   a. Both are process
   b. A, structure; B, outcome
   c. Both are outcome
   d. A, process; B, outcome

4. The nurse manager of the telemetry unit, who reports directly to you, tells you that his unit secretaries are expressing dissatisfactions with their union. They want to vote the union out. You advise that:
   a. Tell the unit secretaries to direct their concerns to their union steward.
   b. Advise them of the procedure for voting the union out.
   c. Ask the manager of labor relations to interview the unit secretaries to document their complaints.
   d. Inform the unit secretaries that management cannot advise the union secretaries on the procedure to vote the union out.

5. You are clinical director of the critical care units. On rounds, you meet Mr. J., aged 80 years, who has consented to coronary artery bypass graft surgery scheduled for tomorrow. He is alert and oriented. He says "I am not sure if I should go ahead with this operation." After you explore his concerns with him, he remains uncertain. You decide to:
   a. Contact his surgeon and accompany the surgeon to talk with Mr. J.
   b. Contact the risk manager for advice as to the legal status of Mr. J.'s consent
   c. Reassure Mr. J. that his surgeon's patients have had successful outcomes
   d. Contact the operating room and cancel the surgery

6. Mr. G., aged 70 years, is admitted to your acute care facility for elective surgery. He is alert and oriented. He has an advanced directive, which is placed in his medical record and correctly documented. Mr. G.'s advanced directive:
   a. Replaces informed consent for specific procedures
   b. Authorizes a health care representative to consent to treatments and procedures
   c. Takes effect only if Mr. G. becomes incapacitated in decision making
   d. Must be reviewed by the hospital's legal counsel before it can be implemented

7. The case management system of patient care delivery has been critical secondary to:
   a. Insurance companies' demand for quality care
   b. The provision of quality care and efficiency
   c. The interprofessional movement in health care
   d. Coordinating prehospital, inpatient, and posthospital care for a caseload of patients

8. When developing criteria for any nursing standards, it is important to make all standards:
   a. Specific and measurable
   b. Outcome oriented
   c. Normative as compared with empirical
   d. Applicable on all nursing units

9. A nurse manager who reports to you has submitted a variance report in which he states that his unfavorable variance in RN wage and salary is due to increased patient acuity. He did not provide any supporting documentation. You will ask him to review with you the patient classification for the reporting period and:
   a. Assignment sheets for the reporting period
   b. Budgeted staffing plan
   c. Hours and earnings report
   d. Capital budget

10. You are an evening shift nursing supervisor. A medical/surgical unit is staffed as follows:

RN	2
LPN	1
Nursing assistant	2
Unit secretary	1
Census	28
Patient classification: I	= 2
II	= 8
III	= 10
IV	= 8

- Note: IV is the highest level of care required.

   The Licensed practical nurse (LPN) called in sick. If all of the following are possible options (i.e., assuming competency of possible replacements and that conditions will be safe on the unit from which you "pull" a replacement; contracts for agency use are in place), you decide to:
   a. Leave the unit without a replacement
   b. "Pull" an LPN from a low-census/low-acuity unit
   c. Obtain an LPN from a contract agency
   d. "Pull" a nursing assistant from a low-census/low-acuity unit

11. As chief nurse executive, you are implementing a plan to close an underutilized unit in an older wing of the hospital and simultaneously increase bed capacity on a unit in a newer wing. Staff of the unit that is closing will be added to staffing of the unit that is expanding. As a follow-up to announcing the plan 2 weeks ago, you have scheduled a meeting with the combined staff of the units involved. You can **best** facilitate staff buy in to this change by **first:**
   a. Encouraging staff to express what they will miss about their former units
   b. Presenting scheduling policies for the new unit
   c. Showing floor plans and sample materials for the new unit that the nurses can select for their unit
   d. Expressing your reservations about the plan

12. On your rounds as evening shift supervisor, the charge nurse of the surgical unit tells you that she thinks Mr. B.'s pleurovac is not functioning properly. She reports that the resident-on-call responded and advised you that there is nothing wrong with the way the device is functioning. You know that it is not functioning properly. To prevent risk of negligence in this situation and to assure a good patient outcome, you:
    a. Tell her to document the resident's assessment of the situation in the medical record; contact the administrator on call
    b. Tell her to document her observations and report the situation to the night charge nurse during the change-of-shift report
    c. Advise her to contact the patient's surgeon
    d. Validate her assessment; contact the resident's immediate supervisor

13. As chief nurse executive, you are reporting to the quality improvement committee of the governing board. You will emphasize how you:
    a. Achieved improvements in patient care
    b. Identified system problems
    c. Resolved difficulties in sampling and data collection
    d. Collaborated with the medical staff to identify and monitor indicators

14. You are deciding whether or not to retain the intravenous therapy team. Which of the following departments will provide the **least** pertinent data?
    a. Finance
    b. Infection Control
    c. Medical Staff Credentialing Committee
    d. Risk Management

15. The nurse manager of the intensive care unit (ICU) reports directly to you. Physicians and managers of other departments have complained to you recently that the ICU nurse manager never seems to be available in the unit when they need him or her to address issues and solve problems. They told you of specific incidents. Your **best** initial response is:
    a. Spend more time in the ICU on your daily rounds to assess the situation
    b. Tell the nurse manager that he or she must increase his or her visibility in the unit
    c. Share the physicians' and managers' perceptions and your concerns about these perceptions with the nurse manager
    d. Ask the nurse manager if he or she has been having any problems lately

16. Most importantly, policies must clearly specify:
    a. Specific steps to be followed by all to whom the policy applies
    b. Objectives to be achieved by enacting the policy
    c. Who is responsible for implementing the policy
    d. Consequences of deviating from the policy

17. The nursing philosophy of the hospital contains:
    a. All components that The Joint Commission requires in the hospital's plan for nursing care
    b. Statements of values and beliefs about nursing, nursing practice, and nursing's role in the organization
    c. Organizational charts and committee structure of the nursing department
    d. Vision, mission, and strategic plan for nursing

18. You are planning to teach your nurse managers how to prepare variance reports in a new format. To **best** apply adult learning principles, you will:
    a. Send a detailed memo including instructions and examples
    b. Demonstrate the procedure for the group using PowerPoint slides; ask the nurse managers what questions they have about the new procedure
    c. Prepare a voice thread of you demonstrating the procedure; allow nurse managers to sign out the video
    d. After demonstrating the procedure for the group, instruct the nurse managers to prepare reports using sample printouts and give feedback

19. The National Labor Relations Act Health Care Amendments of 1974 (Public Law 933-360) include special provisions for health care institutions. These provisions are designed to:
    a. Discourage union activity
    b. Extend jurisdiction to all government-operated health care institutions
    c. Avoid interruptions in the care of patients by the 10-day written notice of intent to strike
    d. Expedite agreements by eliminating written notice provisions for collective bargaining

20. To improve nurse-physician collaboration, the chief nurse executive must **first** assure:
    a. Nursing input into medical staff committees
    b. Documentation of all physician complaints
    c. Joint practice and quality improvement committees
    d. Clinical competence and credibility of the nursing staff

21. Which of the following is the standard of nursing practice most useful for monitoring the quality of nursing performance in the addictions treatment center?
    a. The nurse maintains individual competence in nursing practice.
    b. The patient has the right to expect there will be no Health Insurance Portability and Accountability Act violations.
    c. The nurse completes the admission assessment for each patient, including biophysical, psychosocial, environmental, self-care, educational needs, and discharge planning factors, within 24 hours of admission.
    d. The multidisciplinary treatment team meets weekly to discuss patient care.

22. As a chief nurse executive, you are interviewing an applicant for a nurse manager position. You will place yourself at risk for charges of discrimination if you ask the applicant to:
    a. Describe his or her approach to specific problem situations that have occurred on the unit in the past
    b. Respond to any questions that differ from those you are asking other applicants
    c. Provide a recommendation from his or her present employer
    d. Explain his or her general training and experience received while working as a medic in the military

23. The most recent Joint Commission standards for organizational performance improvement reflect:
    a. Involvement of first-line caregivers; interdisciplinary approach
    b. Use of the plan for nursing services; use of databases for benchmarking
    c. Leadership, management, and staff education in quality; thresholds for evaluation
    d. Focus on structure and process indicators; emphasis on systems

24. As chief nurse executive you have assured the chief operating officer that you will eliminate your special program of premium pay for weekend duty (i.e., Baylor plan) in 6 months. You will be most effective in implementing this change if you:
    a. Brainstorm with your nurse managers as a group to identify alternatives to eliminating the plan
    b. Communicate the decision to all nurse managers and staff as soon as possible
    c. Approach nurse managers on a one-to-one basis to determine impact
    d. Announce elimination of the program 30 days before the implementation date

25. The nurse manager of the ICU, who reports to you, tells you that the housekeeping department is providing unacceptable service in the unit. Your **initial** approach will be to:
    a. Call the director of the housekeeping department and express your concerns
    b. Discuss with the director of human resources the possibility of having unit housekeepers report to the nurse manager
    c. Contact the housekeeping supervisor and tell him or her that he or she needs to discipline some of the ICU housekeepers
    d. Advise him or her to clarify his or her expectations with the housekeeping supervisor

26. The major difference between an open system and a closed system is:
    a. Input
    b. Throughput
    c. Outcome
    d. An open system interacts with the environment

27. Mrs. L., RN, a night nurse in the emergency department, has been on a medical leave of absence while receiving treatment for Demerol addiction. She will return to work next week. You will:
    a. Report Mrs. L.'s return to work to the state board of nursing
    b. Temporarily reassign Mrs. L to a day position on a medical unit with a resultant decrease in salary
    c. Return Mrs. L. to her previous position to avoid discrimination charges
    d. Give Mrs. L. a temporary nonpatient care assignment in utilization review or staff development with a resultant decrease in salary

ANSWERS: 1-c, 2-b, 3-d, 4-d, 5-a, 6-c, 7-b, 8-a, 9-a, 10-b, 11-c, 12-c, 13-a, 14-c, 15-c, 16-c, 17-b, 18-d, 19-c, 20-d, 21-c, 22-b, 23-a, 24-b, 25-d, 26-d, 27-a.

APPENDIX

B

Research Questions

1. What type of statistics describes data?
   a. Inferential
   b. Descriptive
   c. *t*-Test
   d. Chi-square
2. What best describes an outcome variable?
   a. Descriptive
   b. Inferential
   c. Dependent variable
   d. Independent variable
3. What is the best example of inferential statistics?
   a. Table
   b. Graph
   c. Pie chart
   d. *t*-Test
4. What is an example of a qualitative research study?
   a. Experimental design
   b. Quasi-experimental design
   c. Cohort study
   d. Ethnographic study
5. Which type of sample must be present for an experimental design?
   a. Random sample
   b. Convenience sample
   c. Snowball sample
   d. Institutional sample

6. What best represents level I evidence?
   a. Qualitative research study
   b. Quasi-experimental research study
   c. Metasynthesis
   d. Rigorous controlled clinical trial
7. Evidence-based studies can best be described as:
   a. Translational research
   b. Experimental design
   c. Quasi-experimental design
   d. Qualitative research
8. What is the independent variable in the following hypothesis statement? "Patients exposed to a new medication to lower blood pressure will have blood pressure readings lower than those of patients not exposed to this medication or any other intervention."
   a. Blood pressure
   b. New medication
   c. Pulse rate
   d. Blood pressure and new medication
9. What do minors of age of understanding sign as consent for a research study?
   a. Research consent form
   b. Assent
   c. Flow chart
   d. Minors of age cannot consent to research
10. A nurse in a medical center proposed conducting a nonintervention study that involved education of nurses. She presented this to the institutional review board. What type of institutional review board would this study most likely follow?
    a. Expedited review
    b. Normal review process
    c. Delayed review
    d. Exempt review

11. You have just read a research article in a professional journal, which reports that implementing shared governance resulted in no significant increase in expenses. You are wondering if you could introduce shared governance with the same result. You are wondering about which characteristic of this research?
    a. Internal validity
    b. External validity
    c. Reliability
    d. Level of significance

12. The independent variable(s) in the research question, "Is the job performance of nurses affected by years of experience or type of educational program" is (are):
    a. Job performance
    b. Salary
    c. Perceived job autonomy
    d. Years of experience or type of educational program

ANSWERS: 1-b, 2-c, 3-d, 4-d, 5-a, 6-d, 7-a, 8-b, 9-b, 10-a, 11-c, 12-d.

Index

Note: Page numbers followed by "f" indicate figures, "t" indicate tables and "b" indicate boxes.

C

F

O

P

T